AMERICAN MEDICAL ASSOCIATION

PROFILES O ADOLESC HEALTH SERIES

Volume 2

Adolescent Health Care: Use, Costs, and Problems of Access

By (alphabetically)

Janet E. Gans, Ph.D.
Margaret A. McManus, M.H.S.
Paul W. Newacheck, Dr.P.H.

© Copyright 1991 by the
American Medical Association

To place a credit card order for volumes in the
AMA Profiles of Adolescent Health Series,
call 1-800-621-8335.

Volume 1: *America's Adolescents: How Healthy
Are They?* (Order No. OP012690)
ISBN 0-89970-385-2 ISSN 1049-7129

Volume 2: *Adolescent Health Care: Use, Costs,
and Problems of Access* (Order No. OP018091)
ISBN 0-89970-413-1 ISSN 1049-7129

THE AMA PROFILES OF ADOLESCENT HEALTH SERIES

This is the second volume in a series that focuses on major issues in adolescent health. The purpose of the AMA Profiles of Adolescent Health Series is to provide a useful set of references for planning, advocacy, teaching, and community education. The series is intended for people who work with or on behalf of adolescents and who want to know more about the state of their health. Although it provides important information on various topics in adolescent health, the series is not a guide to working with individual adolescents. Each volume in the series is arranged in a question and answer format to enable the reader easily to identify information of greatest interest.

TABLE OF CONTENTS

Page

The AMA Profiles of Adolescent Health Series i

Table of Contents ii

List of Figures iv

List of Boxed Inserts v

Editorial Board of the AMA Profiles of Adolescent Health Series vii

Acknowledgments viii

Executive Summary ix

Introduction 1

Chapter 1   **What health services do adolescents use?** 4

    1. What are the physician and hospital use patterns of adolescents? 5

    2. What dental services do adolescents use? 11

    3. What mental health services do adolescents use? 13

    4. What substance abuse services do adolescents use? 17

    5. What reproductive health services do adolescents use? 19

    6. What are the alternative sites where adolescents
       receive health services? 21

Chapter 2   **How well does health insurance cover the needs of
adolescents and their families?** 27

    1. What is the health insurance status of adolescents
       and how has it changed over time? 28

    2. What types of adolescent health services are typically covered
       by private and public health insurance? 35

    3. How well does health insurance protect adolescents and
       their families from both routine and catastrophic expenses? 37

    4. What are the consequences of being uninsured? 43

Chapter 3 | **What are the nonfinancial barriers to health services for adolescents?** 45

1. In what ways does the organization of health care services limit health care use by adolescents? 46

2. What other factors impede adolescents' use of health services? 54

Chapter 4 | **What can be done to improve access to health services for adolescents?** 58

1. What are the major policy options for reducing the number of uninsured and underinsured adolescents? .59

2. What other steps could ensure that adolescents receive needed health care services? 63

LIST OF FIGURES

Page

Chapter 1 Adolescents With Long Intervals Between Physician Visits 6

Most Common Diagnoses From Adolescent Visits to
Office-Based Physicians 7

Age Differences in Visits to Office-Based Physicians 9

Age Differences in Adolescents' Hospital Stays for
Selected Diagnostic Categories 10

Differences in Adolescent Dental Visits by Family Income 12

Age Differences in Diagnoses of Adolescents Hospitalized
for Mental Disorders 15

Adolescents' Reasons for Visits to School-Based Health Centers 23

Chapter 2 Health Insurance Coverage of Adolescents 28

Characteristics of Adolescents Without Health Insurance 29

Characteristics of Adolescents With Public Health Insurance 31

Characteristics of Adolescents With Private Health Insurance 33

Parents' Reasons Why Their Adolescents Lack Insurance 35

The Adolescent Health Dollar 39

Chapter 3 Health Professionals' Assessment of Their Training
in Adolescent Health 48

Adolescents' Willingness to Seek Health Care Depending
on Parental Involvement 52

Topics Adolescents Want to and Actually Discuss
With Physicians 55

Barriers to Care for Sexually Transmitted Diseases 56

LIST OF BOXED INSERTS

Page

Chapter 1

Recommended preventive health care for adolescents 5

Mental health services for adolescents 14

Native American and Alaskan Native Adolescent Mental Health 16

Data on adolescent alcohol and drug treatment 17

Substance abuse programs for adolescents 18

Determining the effectiveness of adolescent alcohol
and drug treatment 18

Physicians' attitudes toward adolescent alcohol use 19

Adolescent males and family planning services 20

Title XX and adolescent pregnancy 21

Highlights of AMA policy recommendations on
school-based health centers 24

AMA model state legislation for studying the health needs
of incarcerated youth 25

Highlights of AMA policy recommendations on the
health care needs of homeless and runaway youth 26

Chapter 2

Public health insurance for adolescents 30

Private health insurance for adolescents 32

The Early and Periodic Screening, Diagnosis,
and Treatment Program 36

Data on adolescent health care charges and expenses 38

Medical expenses of disabled and nondisabled youth 41

Chapter 3   Availability of physicians with specialty training
in adolescent care 47

Barriers to care for disabled adolescents 50

Chapter 4   Public opinion favors increased spending and services for
adolescent health 59

Proposals by organized medicine to improve access
to medical care 60

Comprehensive and coordinated care efforts sponsored
by the Robert Wood Johnson Foundation 63

Local coordinating health councils 64

Highlights of AMA policy recommendations on
confidential care 65

Professional training in adolescent health and
preventive medicine 67

EDITORIAL BOARD OF THE AMA PROFILES OF ADOLESCENT HEALTH SERIES

The scope and content of each volume in the AMA Profiles of Adolescent Health Series are reviewed by a diverse group of professionals with expertise in child and adolescent health. They include members of the research community, federal government agencies, and physicians. The authors gratefully acknowledge their critical contribution to the series but accept all responsibility for the information included in the volume.

ACKNOWLEDGMENTS

This volume is truly a collaborative effort that spans the entire country, from Washington, DC, to Chicago and San Francisco. The authors would like to thank first the federal Maternal and Child Health Bureau (MCJ-063500), and their project officer, Joann Gephart, R.N., M.S.N. The data on insurance and health expenses are based in part on a federally funded grant to improve health insurance coverage of adolescents. We thank Denise Dougherty, Ph.D. and Urvi Thanawala of the Office of Technology Assessment for providing references and other useful information and statistics. We also appreciate the help of Trina Anglin, M.D., of Cleveland Metropolitan Hospital, Janet Chapin, R.N., M.P.H., of the American College of Obstetricians and Gynecologists, and Cheryl Nelson, Ph.D., of the National Center for Health Statistics.

This volume would not have been possible without the continued support and encouragement of William R. Hendee, Ph.D., Vice President for Science and Technology, and Robert C. Rinaldi, Ph.D., Director of the Division of Health Sciences, both of the American Medical Association. Other colleagues at the AMA helped make this volume useful to physicians and other health professionals working with or on behalf of adolescents. The authors appreciate the careful reviews provided by Arthur B. Elster, M.D., Dale A. Blyth, Ph.D., Linda B. Bresolin, Ph.D., John J. Henning, Ph.D., Katherine H. Voegtle, Ph.D., and Marshall D. Rosman, Ph.D. Kelly Towey deserves special thanks for her outstanding work as a research assistant and noteworthy contribution at each phase in the development of the volume.

Yolanda Davis of the American Medical Association deserves special thanks for her tireless search for materials. Thanks to Nicole Netter for her careful and thorough editorial work. Our special thanks also to Donna McGrath, Denise Keller, and David Doty, who were particularly helpful in turning the manuscript into an attractive and visually appealing book.

EXECUTIVE SUMMARY

Adolescent Health Care: Use, Costs, and Problems of Access
Volume Two in the *AMA Profiles of Adolescent Health Series*

As we approach the end of a century that produced dramatic advances in medical science, an unacceptably large number of adolescents still experience health problems that limit their ability to lead full, productive lives. This is true despite significant declines in adolescent deaths and improvements in the life expectancy of children born with a chronic illness or disability. Increasingly, health problems of today's adolescents are being referred to as "social morbidities" because they are often rooted in the social environment or behavior, rather than being biomedical in origin. As noted in *America's Adolescents: How Healthy Are They?* (50):

- Violence and injury account for three of four deaths among 10- to 19-year-olds. More than 3 of 10 adolescents who die are killed in a motor vehicle accident, and half of these involve alcohol.

- The homicide rate has doubled and the suicide rate has tripled among 10- to 14-year-olds during the past 20 years. Homicide is now the leading cause of death among black 15- to 19-year-olds.

- Abuse and neglect among youth under the age of 18 years increased 74% during the past decade. Adolescents experience more abuse and neglect than younger children do.

- In 1988, 6% of 12- to 17-year-olds consumed alcohol daily, 4% used marijuana daily, and 0.5% used cocaine daily.

- Between 1950 and 1985, the birth rate among unmarried adolescents under 20 years of age increased 300% for whites and 16% for blacks. Approximately 2.5 million adolescents have had a sexually transmitted disease (STD), and one in four sexually active adolescents will have an STD before graduating from high school.

- It is estimated that 5 million children and adolescents need mental health services but do not receive them. Mental disorders reportedly affect 634,000 adolescents and account for 32% of disability among 10- to 18-year-olds.

These statistics underscore the importance of assessing how well the current health system meets the needs of adolescents, particularly those at highest risk for health-related problems.

Use of Health Services and Insurance Status

- Access to health services hinges in part on whether adolescents have health insurance. Most adolescents are covered by insurance. Seventy-four percent of adolescents aged 10 to 18 years are covered by private insurance, 9% by public insurance (largely by Medicaid), and 2% by both public and private insurance.

- Most adolescents (72%) have had contact with a physician during the past year, but 14%—4 million adolescents—last saw a physician more than 2 years ago.

- On the average, adolescents have fewer physician visits and a lower hospitalization rate than any other age group. Most adolescent visits are for preventive care and the treatment of acute conditions.

- Despite relatively high overall rates of insurance coverage among adolescents, some groups of adolescents experience serious problems with access to health care. Uninsured adolescents are at greatest risk for not receiving needed health services. Impoverished, incarcerated, homeless, and minority adolescents are at especially high risk of being uninsured and, therefore, are limited in their access to health services.

Problems of Access

- *Lack of insurance coverage*: Fifteen percent of adolescents (4.7 million) are uninsured. Most adolescents obtain health insurance coverage as dependents under their parents' employer-based plans or Medicaid. Uninsured adolescents typically live in families that cannot afford health insurance and in which the parents' employers fail to offer insurance. Uninsured adolescents tend to be in poorer health, wait longer periods of time between physician visits, and are more likely to be hospitalized, which is due in part to delays in seeking medical care on a timely basis. Uninsured adolescents and their families are more likely than other families to have burdensome medical expenses. Disabled adolescents are more likely than nondisabled adolescents to be uninsured or to have substantial limitations in their coverage.

- *Quality of private coverage*: Adolescents with private insurance are generally well covered for traditional medical services, such as hospital care, physician services, and prescription medicines, but are not well insured for preventive services, maternity-related services, and case management. Most private policies also limit inpatient and outpatient mental health and substance abuse treatment services and impose relatively high cost-sharing requirements for those services.

- *Quality of public coverage*: Adolescent Medicaid recipients are generally well covered for traditional medical services, including preventive care. They are less well insured for physical, occupational, and speech therapy, home health services, case management, substance abuse treatment, and non-physician-provided health services.

- *Limited provider reimbursement*: Inadequate reimbursement rates create additional access problems by discouraging physicians from treating adolescents insured through Medicaid or who require mental health screening and counseling, services that typically require a more lengthy visit.

Nonfinancial Barriers to Care

Beyond insurance status, additional barriers to care exist that either deter adolescents from seeking care or detract from the quality of care received. These barriers include the following:

- *Confidentiality*: Adolescents' concerns about whether problems discussed with the provider will remain confidential may keep them from seeking care.

- *Fragmentation and lack of coordination*: Lack of coordination between health providers as well as health and social service agencies can pose special problems for adolescents with a disability or chronic illness and for other high-risk youth who typically have problems that require the involvement of multiple agencies, such as health, mental health, social service, substance abuse treatment, or juvenile justice agencies.

- *Professional training in adolescent health care*: Relatively few physicians receive training in adolescent medicine, and substantial numbers feel that their specialty training did not adequately prepare them to manage the behavior-related problems of adolescents. In addition, health professionals receive little training on primary and secondary preventive services.

- *Provider sensitivity*: Health providers' sensitivity to the developmental issues of adolescents as well as differences in adolescents' cultural backgrounds may affect communication, compliance with prescribed treatment, and overall health outcome.

- *Adolescent fears and inexperience*: Fears of adolescents, their inexperience or inability to recognize when they have a health problem, and lack of information and skills about where to go for help once they are aware that a problem does exist also deter some adolescents from seeking necessary care.

Proposals to Improve Access to Care

The current system of health care financing in the United States leaves one of every seven adolescents without health insurance protection. Many others have insufficient coverage for the services they need. Two changes that build on our existing financing mechanisms and that could significantly alleviate these problems are the adoption of expanded Medicaid eligibility and the expansion of private health insurance.

- *Expansion of Medicaid*: The newly enacted national eligibility cutoff for Medicaid at the federal poverty level will result in 1.9 million uninsured 10- to 18-year-olds becoming eligible for Medicaid by the year 2002. If all newly eligible adolescents enroll in the program, the size of the uninsured adolescent population would be reduced from 15% to 9.5%. If eligibility were set at 200% of the poverty level, 3.4 million uninsured adolescents would become eligible for Medicaid, potentially reducing the uninsured adolescent population to 4.5%.

- *Mandated employer-provided health insurance*: Mandated employer-provided coverage for employees and their dependents would provide coverage for many uninsured adolescents who would not benefit from the expansion of Medicaid because their family income is too high. If employees who worked 30 hours or more per week were included, approximately 2.5 million currently uninsured adolescents would be covered, reducing the uninsured adolescent population from 15% to 6.9%. An additional 200,000 adolescents would be covered if the mandate applied to all employees who worked 18 or more hours per week.

Employer mandates and Medicaid expansions have different effects on the uninsured adolescent population. The employer mandate would benefit adolescents from modest- and middle-income families, while the Medicaid expansion would benefit the poor and near-poor. If Medicaid were set at 200% of the poverty level and employers were mandated to provide coverage for employees working 18 or more hours per week, 99% of adolescents would have coverage. The remaining 1% would be primarily those adolescents who live with parents who are self-employed. For this population, either a Medicaid or private insurance option could be made available.

While it is critical to overcome financial barriers to care, health insurance alone will not ensure that all adolescents receive needed health care. Nonfinancial barriers must also be removed by increasing the coordination of health services, ensuring confidentiality between adolescents and health providers, and training health professionals in the behavior-related problems of adolescents as well as health maintenance and disease prevention. Health education that enables adolescents to make health-promoting decisions and seek necessary care is also required. It is also critical to expand outreach to special underserved populations such as the disabled, homeless, incarcerated, minority, and rural adolescents, and youth who are no longer in school or living at home.

INTRODUCTION

Adolescence is a time of rapid physical and psychosocial growth and development. Adolescents are relatively healthy, with low rates of cancer, hypertension, and other physical disorders. However, an increasing proportion of today's adolescents engage in risk-taking behaviors that threaten their health as well as their potential to become fully productive members of society. Drug abuse and addiction, sexually transmitted diseases, unintended pregnancy, and mental disorders are among the many problems that affect thousands of adolescents and place growing demands on the health care delivery system.

Of course, not all adolescents engage in health-threatening behaviors. All adolescents, however, need regular preventive and primary care to ensure that problems with their physical and emotional development are identified early and receive necessary treatment. The question of whether adolescents receive needed services can be determined by assessing the proportion who receive health care, the types of services used, and barriers to care, including the lack of or insufficient insurance coverage. It is also important to identify particular groups of adolescents who are at greatest risk for not receiving health services. Once patterns of health care use, financing, and barriers to care have been identified, it should be possible to develop solutions that will expand delivery of appropriate health care services to all adolescents.

In some respects, the health care needs of the 5 million uninsured adolescents are similar to those of all uninsured Americans. That is, any initiatives that provide health insurance coverage to all uninsured Americans would benefit uninsured adolescents. However, additional consideration of the scope of benefits, cost-sharing requirements, and types of qualified health professionals is required to ensure that adolescents have adequate access to needed health services, including preventive care, reproductive health, mental health, and substance abuse services. Some of these services may need to be subsidized by the public sector to ensure that adolescents have access regardless of insurance status.

Even if all adolescents were covered by health insurance, other barriers to care would inhibit their use of health services. Concerns over confidentiality, inadequate availability of specialists trained in adolescent health care, and fragmentation of services are some of the factors that may limit health care access to adolescents. Thus, it is also imperative to address nonfinancial barriers to care in an effort to ensure that adolescents receive comprehensive health services.

Overview of the Volume

The purposes of this volume are to examine adolescent use of health services, health care expenses, health insurance status, and nonfinancial barriers to care. In addition, approaches to improving access to health care will be examined. Chapter 1 describes adolescents' use of medical services, including visits to office-based physicians, hospitals, emergency rooms, and school-based clinics, dental services, and services for mental health, substance abuse, and reproductive health. Also examined are the types of medical specialists adolescents see and the major diagnoses resulting from physician visits and hospital stays.

Chapter 2 describes trends in the health insurance status of adolescents in the United States. The chapter profiles the characteristics of privately insured, publicly insured, and uninsured adolescents. Costs of care and the consequences of being uninsured are discussed. Also discussed are total and out-of-pocket health care expenses, with particular attention to the small proportion of adolescents with high expenses.

Chapter 3 reviews barriers to care that are not financial in nature, particularly ways in which the organization of the health services delivery system limits access to care and inhibits coordination of services. Attitudes and behaviors of adolescents that restrict their use of health services are also described. Chapter 4 examines policy alternatives to reduce financial barriers to care. Also examined are other steps that could ensure that adolescents receive the health services they need, such as assured confidentiality, changes in professional training programs, and increased coordination of services.

Definition of Adolescent Age Groups

Adolescence can be divided into different age groups, each of which reflects a different stage of development. In general, throughout this volume, "early" or "young adolescents" refers to youth aged 10 to 14 years. "Older adolescents" refers to youth aged 15 to 18 years.

Some of the barriers to health services for young adults (between 19 and 24 years of age) are similar to those of adolescents. However, the type and magnitude of barriers to health care faced by young adults are also distinct from those of adolescents, and a full discussion of these barriers is beyond the scope of this book. For this reason, young adults are excluded from our analysis.

Data Used in This Volume

Most data in the volume are based on national surveys. When national data were not available, regional or local samples were used and are noted accordingly. Some of the data were developed specifically for this volume. Data on the proportion of youth who visit physicians, the interval between physician contacts, hospital use, and health insurance status come from special tabulations of the 1986 National Health Interview Survey (NHIS). The NHIS is an annual household interview survey designed to provide information on the health of the U.S. population.

Data on health care expenses are derived from special tabulations of the 1980 National Medical Care Utilization and Expenditure Survey (NMCUES) and have been adjusted to reflect 1990 dollars by means of the medical care component of the Consumer Price Index. The NMCUES data include descriptions of the use of various health services and family expenses for those services. The most current data available at the time of publication have been incorporated whenever possible.

It is difficult to gauge precisely how many adolescents obtain all the preventive and treatment services they need. Incomplete data exist on the level of need among adolescents and the degree to which those needs are being met. Unfortunately, data on use and expenditures for health services have only recently begun to appear in the scientific literature, limiting the depth of the discussion possible on this topic.

There are also other limitations in available data on adolescents. For example, age categories differ from one study to the next, and adolescents are often combined into an age category with either younger children or adults. Whenever possible, data presented in this volume refer to the 10- to 18-year-old age range or specific subgroups within that age range. In some instances, data are unavailable for Hispanics, Asian Americans, or Native Americans. The small numbers of these individuals included in national surveys preclude developing reliable estimates for these populations.

1.

What health services do adolescents use?

The nature of health problems experienced by adolescents has changed dramatically over time. Fifty years ago, natural causes accounted for more than twice as many deaths as violence or injury. The opposite is true today. Today's adolescents are also at greater risk for homicide and suicide, abuse and neglect, substance abuse, obesity, sexually transmitted diseases (including HIV infection and AIDS), and unintended pregnancy. Many of these problems require a different array of preventive and treatment services than was needed in earlier years. The availability and use of these services by adolescents are discussed in this chapter.

Like other age groups, adolescents use health services for preventive care, physical illness, mental disorders, and chronic disease. This chapter examines the number of adolescents using physician and hospital services as well as dental, mental health, substance abuse, and reproductive health services. Use of these services is examined in terms of age, sex, race and ethnic background, family income, and type of community in which the adolescent lives. Also examined is the use of services provided in alternative settings, including emergency rooms, school-based health centers, correctional facilities, and centers for homeless adolescents. The purpose of this overview is to provide background information to determine whether the number, type, and quality of services adolescents receive meet their needs.

The questions addressed in this chapter are:

1. What are the physician and hospital use patterns of adolescents?

2. What dental services do adolescents use?

3. What mental health services do adolescents use?

4. What substance abuse services do adolescents use?

5. What reproductive health services do adolescents use?

6. What are the alternative sites where adolescents receive health services?

1. What are the physician and hospital use patterns of adolescents?

Like all age groups, adolescents experience a variety of acute and chronic conditions, some more serious than others. An acute condition appears suddenly and is generally of short duration but severe enough to involve contact with a physician. Strep throat, a broken leg, and urinary tract infection are examples of acute conditions. A chronic condition is one that lasts for a prolonged time (generally at least 3 months) or recurs from time to time. Cancer, asthma, and diabetes are examples of chronic conditions. Examined in this section are the number and frequency of adolescent visits to physicians and hospitals, and differences in physician and hospital use by age, gender, race and ethnicity, family income, region, and type of community. Also examined are the types of physicians adolescents visit and the major diagnoses associated with physician visits and hospital stays.

Number and Frequency of Physician Visits

In 1986, 72% of adolescents aged 10 to 18 years had at least one contact with a physician. On the average, each adolescent had three physician visits during the year, fewer than most other age groups (103).

Fourteen percent of adolescents last had contact with a physician between 1 and 2 years ago, and another 14%—4 million nationwide—last had contact more than 2 years ago (103).

Recommended preventive health care for adolescents

The American Academy of Pediatrics (7), the Institute of Medicine (126), the American Academy of Family Physicians (5), and the U.S. Public Health Service (132) have each developed guidelines for preventive adolescent health visits. Preventive health visits are recommended at least every 2 years for healthy adolescents and more often for adolescents with health or other problems. The content of recommended preventive visits usually includes health education and anticipatory guidance for adolescents and their parents, early detection of disease, and assessment of physical growth and psychosocial development.

Existing guidelines were designed for adolescents who do not have significant physical problems and who are neither at risk for nor currently engaging in health-compromising behaviors. However, current recommendations need to be reevaluated given the high prevalence of health-compromising behaviors among today's adolescents. A greater number of preventive visits clustered around critical events or developmental stages may be necessary.

The AMA supports the periodic evaluation of adolescents as important for the early detection of disease and for the recognition and correction of risk factors that may lead to disease. The content, timing, and frequency of these visits should vary according to environmental and individual variables and the nature of the diseases targeted for a preventive intervention (16).

Adolescents With Long Intervals Between Physician Visits

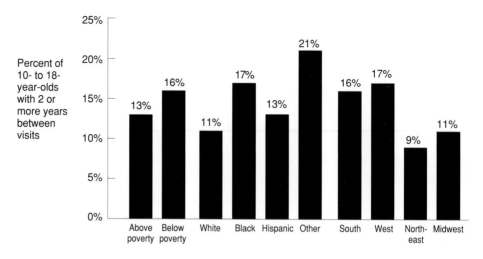

Source: Newacheck, P. W., & McManus, M. A. (1991). Original tabulations from the 1986 National Health Interview Survey.

AMA Profiles of Adolescent Health

◼ Long intervals between physician visits are associated with the family's economic status, race and ethnic background, region of the country, and type of community in which the adolescent lives (103). As shown in the graph:

• Adolescents living in poverty are 1.2 times more likely than nonpoor adolescents to have more than 2 years elapse between physician visits (103).

• Black adolescents are 1.5 times and Hispanic adolescents are 1.2 times more likely than white adolescents to have 2 or more years elapse between physician visits (103).

• Adolescents in the South and West are twice as likely as adolescents in the Northeast to wait 2 or more years between physician visits. Adolescents in the South and West are also more likely

than adolescents in the Midwest to wait more than 2 years between physician visits (103).

Rural adolescents are 1.2 times and adolescents living in the central city are 1.3 times more likely than suburban adolescents to have two or more years elapse between physician visits (103).

Most Common Diagnoses From Adolescent Visits to Office-Based Physicians

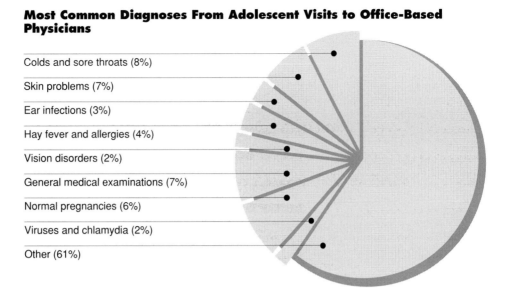

Colds and sore throats (8%)

Skin problems (7%)

Ear infections (3%)

Hay fever and allergies (4%)

Vision disorders (2%)

General medical examinations (7%)

Normal pregnancies (6%)

Viruses and chlamydia (2%)

Other (61%)

Source: Nelson, C. (1991). Office visits by adolescents. In *Advance data from vital and health statistics*, No. 196 (DHHS Publication No. PHS 87-1250). Hyattsville, MD: National Center for Health Statistics.

AMA Profiles of Adolescent Health

Diagnoses From Physician Visits

■ According to the 1985 National Ambulatory Medical Care Survey, office visits made by adolescents to physicians reflect a wide range of specific problems (99). The most common diagnoses for 11- to 20-year-olds are shown in the chart:

• The most common diagnoses are for relatively minor problems. Colds and sore throat, skin problems, ear infections, hay fever and allergy, and vision disorders account for 24% of all adolescent visits (99).

• General medical examinations for preventive care account for 7% of adolescent visits to physicians (99).

• Reproductive health visits for normal pregnancy as well as viruses and chlamydia account for 8% of visits to physicians (99).

• Other diagnoses for adolescent health visits are wide ranging and include various types of injuries and fractures, urinary tract disorders, curvature of the spine and other back problems, anxiety, nervousness, etc. Each accounts for fewer than 2% of visits (99).

Older and younger adolescents have somewhat different diagnoses from visits to office-based physicians. Nine percent of office visits by 15- to 20-year-olds are pregnancy related, compared to fewer than 0.2% of visits by 11- to 14-year-olds. Older adolescents also have more visits than younger adolescents for skin problems, urinary tract disorders, and contraceptive management. Younger adolescents have more visits for general medical examinations, asthma, and curvature of the spine (99).

Adolescent males and females differ in their diagnoses. Sprains, strains, and fractures account for 12% of office-based visits among 15- to 20-year-old males, as do skin problems. Prenatal care accounts for 14% of physician visits by adolescent females, followed by throat problems (9%) (42).

Similar proportions of 11- to 14-year-old boys and girls visit physicians for preventive health examinations (10%) and skin problems (6%), but girls have a higher percentage of visits for coughs and throat problems than do boys (9%) (42).

Types of Physicians Adolescents Visit

Fifty-eight percent of adolescent office visits are to primary care physicians (family practitioners, pediatricians, and internists). Like adults, adolescents also see a variety of other medical specialists. Visits by 11- to 20-year-olds to various types of physicians are as follows:

- 35% of visits are to general and family practice physicians;

- 18% are to pediatricians;

- 8% are to obstetricians and gynecologists;

- 7% are to orthopedic surgeons;

- 6% are to dermatologists;

- 5% are to internists;

- 5% are to ophthalmologists;

- 4% are to general surgeons;

- 3% are to ear, nose, and throat specialists;

- 2% are to psychiatrists;

- 7% are to other specialists, including urologists, neurologists, and others (99).

■ Visits to physicians of various specialties change between early and late adolescence. The percentage of visits by younger and older adolescents are shown in the chart on page 9:

- Between early and late adolescence, visits to a general and family practitioner increase from 31% to 38%, while visits to a pediatrician decline from 33% to 10%. Visits to an obstetrician/ gynecologist increase substantially, from 1% to 10% (99).

- Older adolescents also have twice as many office visits to dermatologists than younger adolescents and 1.5 times more visits to internists or general surgeons (99).

- Visits to psychiatrists account for 2% of office visits by both older and younger adolescents (99).

- Between early and late adolescence, visits to an orthopedic surgeon, ophthalmologist, and ear, nose, and throat specialist decline only slightly (99).

- The other medical specialists adolescents visit include urologists, neurologists, and various other specialists and do not change much between early and late adolescence (7% and 8%, respectively) (99).

Age Differences in Visits to Office-Based Physicians

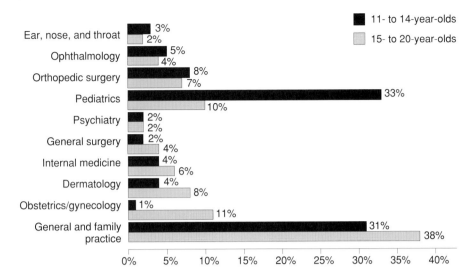

Source: Nelson, C. (1991). Office visits by adolescents. In *Advance data from vital and health statistics,* No. 196 (DHHS Publication No. PHS 87-1250). Hyattsville, MD: National Center for Health Statistics.

AMA Profiles of Adolescent Health

Hospitalization

Consistent with their relatively low prevalence of serious medical disease and chronic illness, adolescents have hospitalization rates below those of other age groups. In 1986, 4% of adolescents between the ages of 10 and 18 years were hospitalized (including maternity). This is less than half the hospitalization rate for the entire U.S. population (9%) (103).

Older adolescents between the ages of 15 and 18 years are more than twice as likely as younger adolescents to have been hospitalized during the past year (5% and 2%, respectively) (103). Age differences in the reasons for hospitalization appear in the following section.

Female adolescents are 1.7 times more likely than males to be hospitalized (5% and 3%, respectively) (103). This is primarily because a

higher percentage of hospitalizations are due to maternity admissions among females (1).

Adolescents living above the poverty level are 1.3 times more likely than adolescents living below the poverty level to be hospitalized (103).

White adolescents are 1.3 times more likely than black adolescents and 1.4 times more likely than Hispanic adolescents to be hospitalized (103).

- It is not clear why white and nonpoor adolescents are more likely to be hospitalized. These differences may be due, in part, to better insurance coverage and more liberal use of hospitalization to treat disease among white and more affluent adolescents.

Adolescents living in rural areas are 1.8 times more likely than those

Age Differences in Adolescents' Hospital Stays for Selected Diagnostic Categories

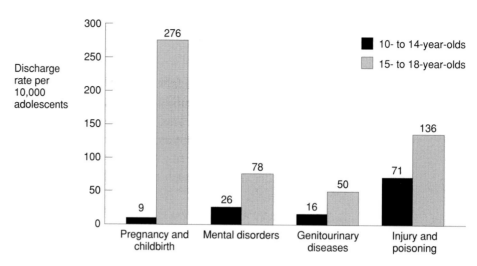

Source: McManus, M., McCarthy, E., Kozak, L. J., & Newacheck, P. (1991). Hospital use by adolescents and young adults. *Journal of Adolescent Health Care, 12,* 107-115.

AMA Profiles of Adolescent Health

in cities, and 1.5 times more likely than suburban adolescents, to be hospitalized (103).

- The higher hospitalization rate and lower rate of physician use among rural adolescents may be due to a lack of accessible primary care, a lack of health insurance, or other factors that delay seeking of medical care until problems are severe enough to require hospitalization (83).

Reasons for Hospitalization

The major reasons for hospitalization among 10- to 18-year-olds are pregnancy and childbirth, injury and poisoning, and mental disorders (82).

◼ Reasons for hospital use among adolescents vary by age and sex, reflecting in large measure the differences in risk-taking behavior.

Age differences in reasons for adolescent hospitalization are shown in the graph:

- The hospitalization rate for pregnancy and childbirth is 30 times greater among older adolescents than younger adolescents (82).

- The hospitalization rate for mental disorders is three times greater among older adolescents than younger adolescents (82).

- The hospitalization rate for diseases of the genitourinary system is also three times greater among older adolescents than younger adolescents (82), most of which reflects the greater prevalence of sexually transmitted diseases among older adolescents.

- The hospitalization rate for injury and poisoning among older adolescents is nearly twice that of younger adolescents (82). Some are alcohol or drug related, and some are attempted suicide (50).

Adolescent boys are more likely to be hospitalized for injury and poisoning, while adolescent girls are more likely to be hospitalized for pregnancy, childbirth, and other obstetrical reasons (82).

Additional information on hospitalization for mental disorders appears in this chapter in question 3, on hospitalization for substance abuse in question 4, and on use of hospital emergency rooms in question 6.

2. What dental services do adolescents use?

Recommended dental care for adolescents consists of both preventive care and routine treatment of acute problems. Hormone changes, poor nutrition, improper hygiene, and genetic predisposition may increase the rate and nature of dental problems that adolescents experience compared to younger age groups. Proper dental care during early adolescence may prevent the shifting of teeth and misalignment or loss of teeth (34) and reduce serious and painful tooth decay, gum disease, and the improper fit between the upper and lower jaws.

Indicators of the increased need for dental services among adolescents include the following:

- Gingivitis, a form of gum disease, increases dramatically between the ages of 12 and 17 years and can result in tooth loss (34).

- Serious tooth decay increases during adolescence from 2% among 12-year-olds to 8% among 17-year-olds (128).

- Malocclusion, the overcrowding and misalignment of teeth due to facial growth, affects half of adolescents (79) and sometimes requires correction through orthodontia.

Seventy percent of adolescents saw a dentist within the past year. However, 73% of white adolescents saw a dentist compared to 59% of Hispanic adolescents and 55% of black adolescents (65).

Differences in Adolescent Dental Visits by Family Income

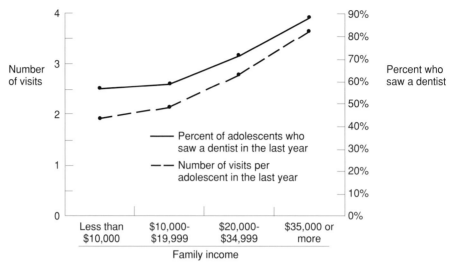

Source: Jack, S., & Bloom, B. (1988). *Use of dental services and dental health, United States: 1986.* Vital and Health Statistics, Series 10, No. 165 (DHHS Publication No. PHS 88-1593). Hyattsville, MD: National Center for Health Statistics.

AMA Profiles of Adolescent Health

■ Adolescents from middle- or upper-income families are more likely to have regular dental care and make more dental visits than adolescents in lower-income families. As shown in the graph:

- Adolescents living in families with an income over $35,000 are 1.5 times more likely to have received dental services during the past year than those whose family incomes are less than $10,000 (65).

- On the average, an adolescent whose family income exceeds $35,000 makes almost twice as many dental visits each year as adolescents whose family income is below $10,000 (65).

Adolescents in middle- or upper-income families usually obtain dental care in private practice settings, while those in low-income families are more likely to use public clinics (52).

Minority adolescents are less likely than whites to receive restorative dental care. By age 17 years, 49% of minority adolescents need fillings compared to 30% of white adolescents (127).

The prevalence of malocclusion is similar across racial and ethnic groups, but treatment rates differ dramatically. Twenty-seven percent of white 17-year-olds receive orthodontic treatment compared to only 4% of nonwhite 17-year-olds (127).

3. What mental health services do adolescents use?

The leading cause of disability among adolescents is mental disorders, including pychoses, anxiety and personality disorders, substance dependence syndromes, and mental retardation. These disorders affect an estimated 634,000 adolescents and account for 32% of chronic conditions among 10- to 18-year-olds (100). Adolescent mental disorders vary in terms of age at onset, type and severity of symptoms, the level of disability they produce, and their long-term effects on development. However, research evidence suggests that many adolescents suffer from two or more mental disorders or have a mental disorder that is complicated by substance abuse or serious delinquency (88).

According to the U.S. Office of Technology Assessment (OTA), at least 7.5 million youth under the age of 18 years (12%) are in need of some type of mental health service, but fewer than one third of those youth actually receive treatment (114).

In 1986, 1.9% (approximately 535,000 10- to 18-year-olds) received care from a mental health facility. Sixty-nine percent used outpatient services, 20% inpatient services, 8% residential treatment centers, and 3% partial hospitalization (33). These figures do not include services provided by private-practice mental health professionals, home-based crisis services, respite care, other residential services such as group homes or therapeutic foster care, or special-ized alcohol and drug treatment facilities.

Outpatient Mental Health Services

Virtually all adolescents who receive outpatient mental health treatment receive evaluation. Fifty-one percent receive individual therapy, 31% family therapy, 10% group therapy, 4% drug therapy, and 4% other types of therapy, such as activity therapy or other rehabilitation (33).

Males are more likely than females to receive outpatient mental health services (54% and 46%, respectively) (33).

Seventy-eight percent of adolescents using outpatient psychiatric services are white and 22% are nonwhite (33), similar to the racial and ethnic composition of the adolescent population in general.

Partial Hospitalization/Day Treatment

Nationally, most adolescents in day treatment have a diagnosed adjustment, behavior, or affective disorder, and 10% are diagnosed with a substance abuse disorder (124).

Adolescent males are three times more likely than females, and whites are more than twice as likely as nonwhites, to use partial hospitalization (33).

Residential Treatment Centers (RTCs)

In 1986, 44,000 adolescents were admitted to residential treatment centers. Males were twice as likely

Mental health services for adolescents

Adolescent mental disorders vary in their severity, their duration, and the therapeutic services necessary to treat them. Wide consensus exists that a continuum of well-integrated, community-based services benefits adolescents' mental health. In 1978 the President's Commission on Mental Health found that few communities provide the amount or range of services necessary to meet the mental health needs of children and adolescents. In many communities this is still the case, with adolescents placed in unnecessarily restrictive settings because less restrictive settings are either unavailable or not covered by health insurance. Listed below is a continuum of mental health treatment services for adolescents, ranging from the least to the most expensive and restrictive (124).

Outpatient care: Adolescents who use outpatient care usually live with their families and do not require 24-hour supervision or partial hospitalization. Outpatient services may be offered in a hospital, clinic, mental health center, private office-based practice, publicly funded clinic, school-based health center, emergency room, crisis center, or therapeutic foster care. (Home-based treatment and hot lines may also be considered outpatient services, but most national data on outpatient mental health care include only visits to a hospital, clinic, mental health center, or private office-based practice [124]).

Partial hospitalization/day treatment: Adolescents who use these services are able to live at home and commute to a structured, therapeutic setting for 4 to 8 hours per day. A less costly alternative to institutional or inpatient care, partial hospitalization typically provides a range of treatment modalities (individual and group therapy, rehabilitation, and, in some instances, academic instruction) (124).

Residential treatment centers (RTCs): RTCs provide 24-hour supervision with limited psychiatric or nursing care. They usually serve patients who are not disturbed enough to be hospitalized or who are already stabilized in their treatment, but not sufficiently stabilized to return to their home environment. RTCs are not licensed as psychiatric hospitals (124).

Inpatient services: These services take place in the psychiatric inpatient unit in a state or county hospital, general hospital, or private psychiatric hospital. Patients usually suffer from severe cognitive, behavioral, and/or affective disorders that keep them from functioning independently at home, at school, or in the community. Psychiatric hospitals provide special diagnostic services, stabilize medication regimens, and use other therapeutic treatments that are sometimes unavailable in less restrictive settings (124).

as females and whites were twice as likely as nonwhites to receive care in a residential treatment center. Minority adolescents are more likely to use RTCs or partial hospitalization than either inpatient or outpatient services (33).

Almost half of the children and adolescents who use residential treatment have a history of inpatient care (121). Detailed diagnoses for children and adolescents who use RTCs are not available.

Inpatient Psychiatric Hospitalization

In 1986, a total of 107,389 10- to 17-year-olds (fewer than 0.5%) were admitted to a hospital for a psychiatric condition. Forty-eight percent were admitted to a general hospital psychiatric unit, 39% to a private psychiatric hospital, and 13% to a state or county psychiatric hospital (33).

Inpatient psychiatric rates for male and female adolescents are very similar; 51% are male and 49% female (33).

Fifteen- to 18-year-olds are more likely than 10- to 14-year-olds to be hospitalized for a mental disorder (31 and 10 per 10,000 adolescents, respectively) (82).

In 1987, 39% of 10- to 18-year-olds hospitalized for a mental disorder were diagnosed as having a psychosis, neurosis, or personality disorder; 18% with alcohol and drug dependence and abuse; 29% with adjustment reaction and disturbance of conduct not elsewhere classified; and 14% with other diagnoses (82).

Age Differences in Diagnoses of Adolescents Hospitalized for Mental Disorders

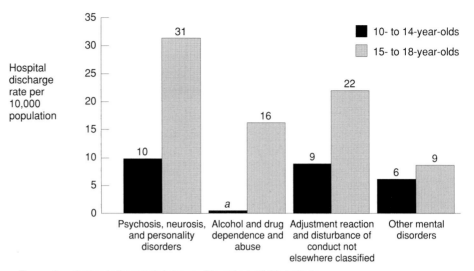

a. The number of cases in the sample is too small to make a reliable estimate.

Source: McManus, M., McCarthy, E., Kozak, L. J., & Newacheck, P. (1991). Hospital use by adolescents and young adults. *Journal of Adolescent Health Care, 12,* 107-115.

AMA Profiles of Adolescent Health

■ The diagnosis for adolescents hospitalized with a mental disorder changes dramatically between early and late adolescence. As shown in the chart:

• The diagnosis of psychosis, neurosis, or personality disorder among adolescents hospitalized with a mental disorder more than triples, from 10 per 10,000 10- to 14-year-olds to 31 per 10,000 15- to 18-year-olds (82).

• The diagnosis of alcohol and other drug dependence and abuse disorder increases from a number too small to make a reliable estimate among 10- to 14-year-olds to 16 per 10,000 adolescents between the ages of 15 and 18 years (82).

• The diagnosis of adjustment reaction and disturbance of conduct more than doubles, from 9 per 10,000 10- to 14-year-olds to 22

per 10,000 15- to 18-year-olds (82).

• The number of other mental disorders diagnosed among hospitalized adolescents shows a smaller increase, from 6 per 10,000 10- to 14-year-olds to 9 per 10,000 15- to 18-year-olds (82).

These estimates should be interpreted with caution because diagnostic patterns may reflect many factors, including differences in the diagnostic and testing criteria used, and reimbursement for certain conditions. In addition, more than one diagnosis may exist per hospital episode. Only the primary diagnosis is discussed in this section.

Between 1980 and 1986, adolescent admissions to psychiatric hospitals increased 33% (33). This trend has generated a great deal of controversy. Critics argue that some parents place their adolescents in hospitals because their communities lack a continuum of mental health services and because insurance primarily covers inpatient services (38, 115).

Factors contributing to the controversial increase in the psychiatric hospitalization of adolescents, particularly in private psychiatric hospitals, include a shift away from the use of state and county mental hospitals, divorce or family disruption, decreased stigma of psychiatric treatment, and insurance policies that reimburse for inpatient services rather than less expensive, outpatient services (38, 115).

Native American and Alaskan Native adolescent mental health

According to a 1990 report by the Office of Technology Assessment, Native American adolescents have more serious mental health problems than other groups in the United States. These problems include mental retardation and learning disabilities, depression, suicide, anxiety, alcohol and substance abuse, self-esteem and alienation, running away, and dropping out of school. For example, the suicide rate is 160% higher among Native Americans and Alaskan Natives than other groups in the United States, and their school dropout rate is estimated as being between 2 and 3 times greater.

Approximately 400,000 children and adolescents live in Indian Health Service areas, but limited funds allow only for a ratio of less than 1 mental health provider to every 20,000 children and adolescents. Virtually no alcoholism services are designed for Native American adolescents, and little coordination or continuity of care exists among alcohol, social service, and mental health programs (78). The OTA urges the expansion of community-based, comprehensive mental health services for Native American and Alaskan Native adolescents, emphasizes that the expansion should be sensitive to their particular cultural needs, and underscores the need for coordination among service agencies (78).

Although the majority of adolescent admissions to private psychiatric hospitals may be appropriate, the National Institute of Mental Health (NIMH) estimates that community-based outpatient or residential settings could effectively treat as many as 40% of the children and adolescents who currently receive care in more expensive, inpatient settings (97). The factors that affect the effectiveness of different psychiatric treatments are complex and vary depending on the individual patient (50).

It appears that specialized treatment and aftercare services can ease the transition to the family or community, thereby enhancing the effectiveness of adolescent inpatient psychiatric hospitalization. Adolescent inpatient psychiatric treatment is more effective among less severely disturbed adolescents than among the more severely disturbed. Length of stay and IQ have a moderate, positive impact on patient outcome, but age at admission and sex of the patient have little effect (110).

Although more adolescents today receive mental health services, the vast majority in need do not. Minorities and adolescents from low-income families are even less likely to receive mental health services than are white adolescents and adolescents living in middle- and upper-income families. Shortages in mental health services are especially acute for community-based services, case management, and coordination across child service systems (114).

4. What substance abuse services do adolescents use?

Since the 1950s, adolescents have tried alcohol and other substances at progressively younger ages. Some of those who experiment with alcohol or drugs eventually suffer serious physical, mental, and/or social consequences and require treatment. This section examines the number of adolescents who participate in alcohol and drug treatment programs that are funded, at least in part, by state funds. Data for alcohol and drug treatment are presented separately, though some adolescents participate in programs that treat abusers of both alcohol and drugs.

Data on adolescent alcohol and drug treatment

Information about drug and alcohol treatment in the United States is very limited, especially for adolescents. The best national data come from the National Drug and Alcoholism Treatment Unit Survey (NDATUS), which is conducted by the National Institute on Drug Abuse (NIDA) and the National Institute on Alcohol Abuse and Alcoholism (NIAAA). However, NDATUS data fail to differentiate between children and adolescents. Descriptions of the type of treatment received, funding sources and amounts, and staffing patterns are also not reported by age, which limits the picture of adolescents' use of substance abuse services. In addition, the data reported by NDATUS include patients enrolled in an alcohol or drug treatment program during a 1-month period; estimates are not for the entire year (95).

Adolescent substance abuse may precede, coincide with, or result from poor school performance, school dropout, difficulty with family and peer relationships, delinquency, injury, and emotional or mental disorders (40). Many substance-abusing adolescents come from families in which one or both parents abuse alcohol or other sub-

stances. A recent survey found that 55% of adolescents receiving inpatient substance abuse treatment reported having a family member who engaged in excessive drinking, and 32% reported excessive drug use by a family member (55).

In 1987, approximately 272,000 adolescents (1%) were treated for abuse of alcohol or other substances (124).

Only 10% of adolescents who drank alcohol excessively were in alcohol treatment. Approximately 157,000 adolescents were in alcohol treatment (124), though approximately 1.1 million 12- to 17-year-olds drank alcohol daily (96).

Only as many as 20% of adolescents who smoked marijuana daily were in drug treatment programs. That year approximately 783,000 adolescents smoked marijuana daily (96), but only 157,000 were in drug treatment programs for all substances (124).

Adolescents account for 6% of the total U.S. population being treated for alcohol abuse and 15% of those being treated for drug abuse (105).

Approximately 18% of drug treatment programs serve adolescents only. These programs serve nearly half of all adolescents in treatment (105).

Substance abuse programs for adolescents

Substance abuse programs for adolescents fall into one of three general categories: (1) prevention programs that seek to deter or delay the use of alcohol and other licit and illicit substances, (2) assessment or referral services in which the goal is to identify whether the individual has a substance abuse problem and, if so, to find appropriate resources for treatment, and (3) treatment programs for adolescents with identified substance abuse problems who require intervention because of actual or potential functional impairment. Treatment programs range from inpatient or residential care to less restrictive, outpatient or day treatment programs, or self-help and peer counseling groups (124).

Adolescent substance abuse prevention programs generally occur within the community, usually in schools, youth groups, or other recreation facilities. They typically target younger adolescents who have not yet tried substances or who are just beginning to experiment with them. Treatment programs are usually located outside of the adolescent's community and target older adolescents whose addiction may require residential treatment (124).

Determining the effectiveness of adolescent alcohol and drug treatment

It is difficult to estimate the number of adolescents who need and use alcohol and drug treatment and to gauge the effectiveness of their treatment. A lack of consensus exists regarding the point at which an adolescent should be classified as needing alcohol or drug treatment, the type of intervention required, and the most appropriate type of treatment setting. Little is known about the effectiveness of substance abuse services in terms of the substance involved, whether certain programs are more effective with certain populations, and whether they prevent relapse into abuse or dependence. However, inpatient substance abuse treatment services appear to be most effective with adolescents who . . .

• admit to being chemically dependent (55);

• perceive themselves as having entered treatment voluntarily (28);

• live with at least one parent (55);

• participate in a program that includes family therapy (27).

Substance abuse treatment is less effective among those who have failed in school, began substance abuse at a younger age, use multiple drugs, or have an arrest record. The majority (55%) of adolescents who fail to complete inpatient substance abuse treatment are discharged by staff for noncompliance. The remainder of this group leave treatment against staff advice (55).

More than four out of five adolescents treated for alcohol or substance abuse problems obtain care through an outpatient program (105).

According to the Office of Technology Assessment, family income and insurance status have a substantial impact on the type of alcohol or substance abuse program an adolescent enters. An adolescent from an upper-income family or one who has insurance generally receives more intensive services offered in private settings. An adolescent from a low-income family typically receives public services, which generally have long waiting lists and may be less comprehensive (124).

Males account for two thirds of adolescents in treatment for alcohol abuse and more than half of those in treatment for drug abuse (124).

More substance abuse programs specifically tailored to the unique needs of adolescents are needed. Adolescent substance abuse programs must begin to involve the entire family, not just the adolescent, and should integrate prevention and intervention efforts that target other health problem areas. More research on the effectiveness of prevention and intervention strategies is also needed.

Physicians' attitudes toward adolescent alcohol use

A 1987 survey by the American Medical Association found that 96% of physicians believed that alcohol abuse was a serious problem among adolescents between the ages of 12 and 18 years, and 95% favored health insurance coverage for the treatment of drinking problems and alcoholism. Seventy-three percent of physicians reported having initiated a discussion about alcohol use with adolescent patients, and 57% reported having talked about alcohol use with the parents of these patients. When asked about treatment for an adolescent with an alcohol problem, 57% of physicians said that they would refer the adolescent to a specialized treatment program; 42% said that they would treat the patient in addition to referring the patient to a special program. Seventy-nine percent thought that medical schools should increase the amount of time spent on education about alcohol problems (12).

5. What reproductive health services do adolescents use?

By age 18 years, 51% of girls and 65% of boys in the United States report having had sexual intercourse (85). Two and a half million adolescents have a sexually transmitted disease (50). More than 600 adolescents have AIDS, and thousands are infected with HIV (35). Each year 1 million adolescents get pregnant (an average of 3,000 a day). Of these, 477,000 give birth, more than 400,000 have abortions, and approximately 137,000 have miscarriages (58). These alarming statistics underscore the need for appropriate reproductive health services for adolescents.

In 1988, 30% of 15- to 19-year-old women had a family planning visit for birth control, a pregnancy test, or counseling. Black 15- to 19-year-old women were 1.4 times more likely than white peers to have had a family planning visit (87).

Sixty-two percent of 15- to 19-year-old women who have a family plan-ning visit use a clinic rather than a physician's office, citing lower cost and greater perceived confidentiality as the primary reasons for using a clinic (87).

Fifteen- to 17-year-old women are more likely than 18- to 19-year-old women to use a family planning clinic for their *first* visit (66% and 57%, respectively) (87).

Race differences in adolescent use of family planning clinics have diminished over time, primarily due to a shift among white adolescents from private physicians' offices to family planning clinics. In 1982, black 15- to 19-year-old women were 67% more likely than their white peers to use a clinic rather than a physician's office. In 1988 they were only 6% more likely to use a clinic (87).

Between 40% and 60% of adolescents report that their parents are aware of their use of a family planning clinic (86, 122), and 12% report using the family planning clinic at their parents' suggestion (36).

Abortion Services

Most abortions take place in clinics located in large metropolitan counties. In 1985, only 2% of abortions nationwide took place in rural communities or small towns (58).

Fifteen- to 19-year-olds account for 25% of all abortions. An estimated 4% of 15- to 19-year-old women had an abortion in 1985 (59).

Adolescent males and family planning services

Except for condom distribution programs, males' roles in pregnancy prevention and contraception have been secondary to the efforts targeting females. Adolescent and young adult males are less likely to use family planning clinics or other settings perceived as targeting young women (41). In a survey that asked inner-city males why they did not seek birth control devices from a clinic, 74% said that they were too embarrassed or uncomfortable to ask for a condom, 48% felt uncomfortable using the clinic just for condoms, and 37% did not want to tell the receptionist at the front desk that they wanted a condom, or did not know how to ask for them (111).

In a survey asking women under the age of 18 years why they decided to have an abortion . . .

- 92% were concerned about how a baby would change their life;

- 81% felt too young and immature to have a child;

- 73% reported that they could not afford to have the baby;

- 28% reported that their parents wanted them to have an abortion;

- 23% said that their husbands or partners did not want them to have the baby;

- 37% cited problems with their relationship with the father and did not want to be a single parent (123).

Services for Pregnant and Parenting Adolescents

Pregnant adolescents under the age of 20 years are less likely than women in other age groups to obtain early prenatal care. They are more likely to receive late or no prenatal care (36 weeks of gestation or later) (61).

- Of babies born to adolescents in 1985, 53% had mothers who received care in the first 3 months of pregnancy, compared to 76% of babies born to women of all ages (61).

- In 1985, 6% of babies were born to women of all ages who received late or no prenatal care, compared to 12% of babies born to adolescents (61).

Only 4% of unmarried adolescent mothers offer their babies for adoption (3), and the use of adoption services appears to be declining over time.

- Between 1969 and 1985, the number of member agencies of the Child Welfare League of America (CWLA) offering adoptive placement declined from 97% to 63%. In 1985, only 26%

Title XX and adolescent pregnancy

In 1981 Congress enacted the Adolescent Family Life Act, under Title XX of the Public Health Service Act. This program mandates funds for pregnancy and parenting services to be administered through the Office of Adolescent Pregnancy Programs in the Office of Population Affairs (OPA). The OPA is also responsible for administering federal family planning funds under Title X of the Public Health Service.

Title XX funds are intended for model programs that directly provide or coordinate a set of specific, comprehensive services for pregnant adolescents, their infants, and their families. Title XX legislation mandates that a portion of the funds be used for program evaluation and for research about issues pertinent to adolescent pregnancy, such as adoption and prevention. Use of Title XX funds for abortion and abortion counseling is prohibited. Since Title XX was enacted, 77 care projects involving health education and social services, 54 prevention projects that promote abstinence, and 10 projects combining care and prevention have been funded and include most states and U.S. territories (107).

of CWLA agencies listed adoption among their top five services used by adolescents (119, 133).

Residential placement for pregnant and parenting adolescents has recently increased after a long period of decline (53). Approximately 33% of member agencies of the CWLA offer prebirth residential or group home care, but only 18% offer postbirth residential care (133).

6. What are the alternative sites where adolescents receive health services?

Certain adolescents have difficulty gaining access to health services. These adolescents may have at least some of their health needs met by emergency rooms and school-based health centers. Homeless and incarcerated youth are much more likely to go without health and social services, placing them at great risk for a wide variety of health problems. Adolescents with chronic illnesses are also at risk for being underserved.

Emergency Room Services and Public Clinics

Although emergency rooms were established for the treatment of urgent problems, they have been used increasingly for the treatment of minor illnesses, particularly among racial and ethnic minorities, those who lack either a regular physician or health insurance, and those who

are unaware of alternative health care options (135).

Approximately one in seven 12- to 17-year-olds receives routine medical care from a public hospital outpatient clinic, hospital emergency room, walk-in or emergency care center, or another public clinic or health center. Adolescents who receive care from one of these settings tend to come from a low-income family, belong to a racial or ethnic minority, and lack health insurance (29).

• Adolescents whose family income is less than $10,000 are almost 5 times more likely than adolescents whose family income exceeds $40,000 to receive regular medical care from a public clinic (29).

- Black adolescents are 3.3 times and Hispanics 2.5 times more likely than white adolescents to receive routine care from public clinics (29).

- Adolescents without health insurance are 2.5 times more likely than insured adolescents to receive regular medical care from public clinics (29).

Little is known about the medical reasons for adolescents' use of emergency rooms. A survey of free-standing emergency centers in Houston found that 41% of adolescents came for general medical examinations. Thirty-six percent came for trauma-related causes, such as wounds, lacerations, bruises, burns, sprains, fractures, and other injuries (138).

Some adolescents use emergency rooms for substance abuse-related crises. The most comprehensive national data on substance-related emergency room visits come from the Drug Abuse Warning Network (DAWN) system, which is composed of 770 emergency rooms in 27 U.S. cities and 87 medical examiners in 27 cities (94).

In 1989, 12,611 adolescents between the ages of 10 and 17 years went to an emergency room in the DAWN system with a substance abuse-related problem. Of these visits . . .

- 76% had overdosed on a drug;

- 4% sought detoxification or were experiencing withdrawal;

- 2% had experienced an accident or injury while using drugs;

- 18% sought care for other substance-related reasons (94).

Sixty-three percent of adolescent drug-related emergency room visits involved the use of a single drug, and 36% involved more than one drug (other than alcohol). Sixty-five percent of adolescent drug-related emergency room visits appear to be suicide related (94).

Most adolescent substance-related visits to the emergency room involved legal substances that are used without medical approval. Alcohol in combination with other drugs accounts for 13% of DAWN-reported drug abuse. Ibuprofen, acetaminophen, codeine, over-the-counter sleep aids, caffeine, and over-the-counter diet pills are some of the drugs most commonly related to adolescent emergency room visits in the DAWN system (94).

School-Based Health Centers

School-based health centers were originally developed to increase access to primary health services, especially for low-income, nonwhite, and rural adolescents. Currently more than 150 school-based health centers in 32 states provide services to adolescents who might not otherwise receive needed care (62).

Controversy surrounding school-based health centers revolves around reproductive health services, particularly the distribution of contraceptive devices or prescriptions. However, only 20% of total visits to these school-based health programs are for family planning services (17), and only 15% of school-based health centers dispense contraceptives (76).

Adolescents' Reasons for Visits to School-Based Health Centers

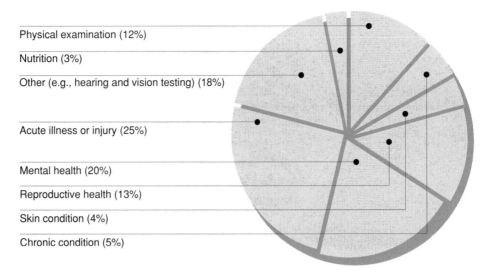

Physical examination (12%)

Nutrition (3%)

Other (e.g., hearing and vision testing) (18%)

Acute illness or injury (25%)

Mental health (20%)

Reproductive health (13%)

Skin condition (4%)

Chronic condition (5%)

Source: Lear, J. G. (1989). *The school-based adolescent health care program.* Proceedings from the 1989 Adolescent Health Coordinators Conference. Washington, DC: National Center for Education in Maternal and Child Health.

AMA Profiles of Adolescent Health

Most school-based health centers offer the following array of services: primary medical health services, assessment and referral to a community health care center or a community physician, sports physical assessment, general physical examination, laboratory testing, diagnosis and treatment of minor trauma, and prescribed medications (76).

A majority of school-based health centers also provide more specialized services that include health and nutrition education, mental health and psychosocial counseling, sexuality counseling (including gynecologic examinations, pregnancy diagnosis, counseling, and referral for antenatal care), and weight reduction programs (76).

■ The primary diagnoses made by school-based clinics (based on more than 47,000 adolescent visits) appear below:

• Preventive care for physical examinations, nutrition counseling, and hearing and vision testing account for 33% of visits to school-based health centers (72).

• Acute illness, injury, and mental health problems account for 45% of visits, more than 3 times as many visits as for reproductive health (72).

In 1989, almost 80% of students enrolled in their school-based health center used services provided by the school-based center at least once during the academic year. More than half of these students report having no other source of primary health care (69).

In 1988, males constituted 38% of those who used a school-based health center, a higher percentage than the percentage who used other nontraditional health delivery systems (76).

School-based health centers appear to hold great promise for the delivery of basic and specialized health services to adolescents who might not otherwise receive care. Despite their promise, however, school-based health centers will still not reach adolescents who have matriculated or those who have

dropped out of school. They typically provide care only during the school day and year and tend to have a limited capacity for secondary and tertiary care. Lack of stable funding sources adversely affects the continuity of care in some programs (17).

Health Services in Correctional Institutions

Each year approximately 500,000 children and adolescents are admitted to juvenile detention facilities, and another 500,000 are kept in adult jails or lockup facilities (6). Incarcerated adolescents represent a vastly underserved population with greater than average health care needs. Many have underlying, undiagnosed, or untreated physical and emotional disorders, and most lack a coordinated source of regular health care (15).

Approximately 20% of juveniles in correctional facilities currently meet or have in the past met diagnostic criteria for major depression (15), and 63% used drugs regularly before their incarceration. Thirty-two percent were under the influence of alcohol and 39% were under the influence of another drug when they committed their offenses (84). Ten percent were classified as neglected, abused, emotionally disturbed, or mentally retarded (129).

The small amount of data on the health care provided to incarcerated adolescents comes from local or regional surveys of juvenile detention centers, and much of this information is dated (57, 67). A 1983 survey of juvenile facilities

---

Highlights of AMA policy recommendations on school-based health centers

The AMA recognizes the promise of school-based health centers to provide health services to adolescents, particularly in medically underserved areas. Where school-based health services exist, they should meet the following minimum standards: (a) Health services in schools must be supervised by a physician, preferably one who is experienced in the care of children and adolescents. Additionally, a physician should be accessible to administer care on a regular basis. (b) On-site services should be provided by a professionally prepared school nurse or similarly qualified health professional. Expertise in child and adolescent development, psychosocial and behavioral problems, and emergency care is desirable. Responsibilities of this professional would include coordinating the health care of students with the student, the parents, the school, and the student's personal physician and assisting with the development and presentation of health education programs in the classroom. (c) There should be a written policy to govern provision of health services in the school, developed by a school health council consisting of school and community-based physicians and nurses, school faculty and administrators, parents and (as appropriate) students, community leaders, and others. (d) Before patient services begin, policies on confidentiality should be established with the advice of expert legal advisors and the school health council. (e) Policies for ongoing monitoring, quality assurance, and evaluation should be established and executed. (f) Health care services should be available during school hours. During other hours an appropriate referral system should be instituted. (g) School-based health programs should draw on outside resources for care, such as private practitioners, public health and mental health clinics, and mental health and neighborhood health programs. (h) Services provided should be coordinated to ensure comprehensive care. Parents should be encouraged to be intimately involved in the health supervision and education of their children (17).

conducted by the National Commission on Correctional Health Care found that only:

- 83% provide a regularly scheduled sick call;

- 60% provide medical screening when first admitted to the facility to detect medical or mental problems that require immediate attention;

- 72% provide a physical examination within the first week of a juvenile's admission;

- 49% provide ongoing mental health services;

- 58% provide ongoing dental services (24).

Sixteen percent of juvenile incarceration facilities report at least one death during the past 5 years. Sixty-four percent of the reported deaths were by suicide (24).

In general, smaller juvenile correctional facilities offer less adequate health services than larger facilities do (24).

Health Services for Homeless Adolescents

An estimated 500,000 homeless adolescents live in the United States (14). Their lifestyles place them at high risk of violence and injury, substance abuse, sexual abuse, sexually transmitted diseases including AIDS, malnutrition, and other health problems. Therefore, they are likely to have serious unmet needs for health and other social services. It is a major challenge for the current health care system to deliver comprehensive services to a population with such complex health problems.

Issues of reimbursement, consent, and confidentiality, as well as the ambiguous legal status of minors, frequently preclude prompt and full treatment of homeless and runaway youth. Many homeless youth distrust authority figures and put off seeking care until problems become so severe that they can no longer be postponed (14).

AMA model state legislation for studying the health needs of incarcerated youth

In 1990, the AMA Board of Trustees approved a model state bill to create a blue-ribbon panel to study the physical and mental health care needs of detained and incarcerated youth and to make recommendations for further legislation. The panel would consider specific preexisting health problems as well as health problems associated with incarceration (e.g., problems of self-inflicted injury, accidental injury, excessive weight gain, physical and sexual abuse, and suicidal behavior). They would also consider the health care standards specific for juvenile corrections institutions established in 1979 by the AMA and later revised by the National Commission on Correctional Health Care: regularly scheduled sick call by a qualified health professional, an initial medical screening performed by a qualified health professional or health-trained staff, a complete health appraisal within the first 7 days of admission, a dental screening within the first 7 days, dental hygiene services within the first 14 days, a dental examination within the first month, ongoing dental services, and ongoing mental health services. The blue-ribbon panel would also consider problems of excessively aggressive play often encouraged by institutional staff, overcrowding, the management of poor behavior, overuse of isolation and chemical or mechanical restraints, side effects produced by psychotropic medications, and the stress of close containment.

The panel would consult with organizations having particular expertise on the topic, including the National Commission on Correctional Health Care, the National Association of Juvenile and Family Court Judges, the American Correctional Association, the American Medical Association, the American Academy of Pediatrics, and the American Academy of Child and Adolescent Psychiatry. It would issue a comprehensive report to the governor and to the State House of Representatives and Senate (11).

It is important that health care providers treat homeless and runaway youth in a nonjudgmental and nonthreatening manner and, insofar as possible, provide comprehensive treatment during the initial visit, because many of these adolescents do not return for follow-up care (14).

Health Services for Disabled Adolescents

Nearly 2 million 10- to 18-year-olds (6%) suffer from some degree of limitation in their activities due to a chronic condition. The prevalence of disability is similar among adolescents of different racial and ethnic groups. However, adolescents living in a family below the poverty level are 1.4 times more likely to have an activity limitation than those in a family above the poverty level (100).

Disabled adolescents average eight physician visits per year, three times as many as nondisabled adolescents. Disabled adolescents are also nearly five times more likely than nondisabled adolescents to be hospitalized and, on the average, spend twice as many days per hospital stay (100).

The costs of health services for disabled adolescents are discussed in the following chapter. Barriers to health services for disabled adolescents are discussed in chapter 3.

Summary and Implications

Changes in the nature of adolescent health problems during the past 20 years, particularly the increase in the "social morbidities," have produced a need for different and expanded health services that focus on both prevention and intervention. The range and number of health care services adolescents use depend on various factors, such as family income, health insurance coverage, geographic location, and the race and ethnic background of the adolescent. While some adolescents have been able to get the health services they need, others have not. For poorer, uninsured, and out-of-school adolescents, alternative health care providers such as school-based health centers, adolescent clinics, and family planning clinics may help meet certain needs.

Highlights of AMA policy recommendations on the health care needs of homeless and runaway youth

Medical care for homeless and runaway adolescents is generally inadequate for reasons that include a shortage of facilities, the serious health-threatening behaviors of these adolescents, the inability of health professionals to deal with such youth, legal complications of providing treatment, and the dearth of treatment guidelines. Data on the extent of homelessness among adolescents is sorely lacking, and little is known about the health needs and services provided to the adolescent homeless population. In view of these facts, the American Medical Association has made the following recommendations: (a) Funding should be provided by an appropriate government agency for a national study that would provide accurate, timely, and reliable data on homeless adolescents. (b) Consider conducting a pilot study of the health care needs of homeless youths in a major city to provide physicians with solid baseline data on this issue. (c) Explore the feasibility of establishing a protocol to be used in the evaluation and treatment of homeless youths. (d) Disseminate information on the lack of treatment facilities and health care providers for treating homeless youths. (e) Encourage state medical societies to determine the extent of treatment possible under state law, to inform physicians of the laws and regulations affecting the treatment of minors, especially those who are homeless, and to form linkages with statewide youth advocacy groups to develop protocols for the treatment of troubled youths. (f) Encourage local medical societies to develop and publicize lists of local and regional resources that can assist homeless adolescents, to provide this information to local physicians, and to establish links with providers of youth services to improve knowledge of the needs and limitations of these youth and physicians who provide care (14).

Chapter

2.

How well does health insurance cover the needs of adolescents and their families?

As described in chapter 1, adolescents use a broad array of health care services. This chapter examines the health insurance status of adolescents and the critical role that coverage plays in whether an adolescent obtains needed medical services. It also examines changes in the insurance status of adolescents over time as well as the reasons why some adolescents lack health insurance. The costs of adolescent health are examined in terms of overall costs and the expenses families pay out of pocket.

The adequacy of health insurance for adolescents is explored in terms of the scope and duration of services typically covered and the degree to which coverage protects adolescents and their families from catastrophic expenses. The chapter concludes with a discussion of the consequences of being uninsured or underinsured, which occurs when a policy fails to cover necessary services or does not cover substantial medical costs.

The questions addressed in this chapter are:

1. What is the health insurance status of adolescents and how has it changed over time?

2. What types of adolescent health services are typically covered by private and public health insurance?

3. How well does health insurance protect adolescents and their families from both routine and catastrophic expenses?

4. What are the consequences of being uninsured?

Health Insurance Coverage of Adolescents

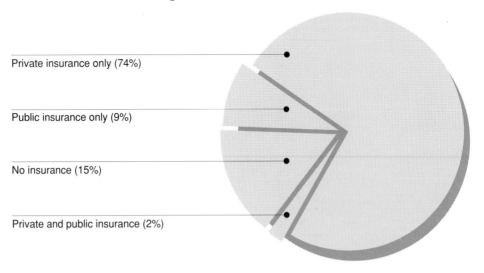

Private insurance only (74%)

Public insurance only (9%)

No insurance (15%)

Private and public insurance (2%)

Source: Newacheck, P. W., & McManus, M. A. (1991). Original tabulations from the 1986 National Health Interview Survey.

AMA Profiles of Adolescent Health

1. What is the health insurance status of adolescents and how has it changed over time?

Most adolescents are covered by private or public health insurance, depending on the insurance status of their parents. Parents' coverage, in turn, is usually a function of their employers' insurance packages or eligibility for public insurance. This section examines the health insurance status of adolescents and changes in the uninsured adolescent population during the past decade.

◼ As shown in the chart:

• The vast majority (85%) of adolescents between the ages of 10 and 18 years are covered through either private or public health insurance (103).

• Seventy-four percent of adolescents are privately insured, 9% are publicly insured, and 2% are covered through both private and public sources (103).

• As many as 4.7 million adolescents (15%) are without health insurance protection (103).

Characteristics of Adolescents Without Health Insurance

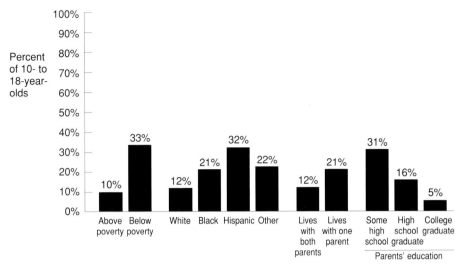

Source: Newacheck, P. W., & McManus, M. A. (1991). Original tabulations from the 1986 National Health Interview Survey.

AMA Profiles of Adolescent Health

Characteristics of Uninsured Adolescents

■ Adolescents without health insurance typically live in poverty or near poverty and with a parent whose job does not include health insurance benefits. Many live in single-parent families and have parents with little education. As shown in the graph:

• Adolescents living in poverty are 3.3 times more likely to be uninsured than those not in poverty (103).

• Black adolescents are 1.8 times and Hispanics 2.8 times more likely to be uninsured than white adolescents (103).

• Adolescents living with one parent are 1.7 times more likely to be uninsured than those living with both parents (103).

• Adolescents whose parents never graduated from high school are

nearly twice as likely to be uninsured as those whose parents graduated from high school. Adolescents whose parents graduated from high school are 3.2 times more likely to be uninsured than those whose parents graduated from college (103).

Geographic and age differences also exist between insured and uninsured adolescents. Adolescents in the South or West are twice as likely to be uninsured as adolescents living in the Northeast or Midwest (103).

Uninsured adolescents are more likely to reside in the central city (19%) or a rural area (18%) than in the suburbs (12%) (103).

Fifteen- to 18-year-olds are 1.2 times more likely to be uninsured than 10- to 14-year-olds (103).

Public health insurance for adolescents

Public health insurance includes Medicaid, Medicare, and the Civilian Health and Medical Program of the Uniformed Services (CHAMPUS). Medicaid is the largest federal public health program for children and adolescents in low-income families and has played an important role in reducing the disparity in access to care between the poor and nonpoor (113). It entitles eligible, poor individuals to a range of medical benefits, with the federal government reimbursing states for a portion of the incurred costs on the basis of a formula tied to a state's per capita income level. Historically, enrollment in the Medicaid program has been tied to eligibility for public assistance programs, including Aid to Families With Dependent Children (AFDC) and the Supplemental Security Income (SSI) program for the disabled. Until recently, a family with an adolescent generally had to qualify for AFDC or SSI cash assistance before obtaining Medicaid coverage. This link has recently eroded for children and adolescents below the federal poverty level with Medicaid expansions in the late 1980s and 1990.

Once enrolled in Medicaid, adolescents are covered for basic health care services, including hospital care and physician services, without the deductibles and coinsurance common to private health insurance plans. However, it can be difficult for adolescents covered by Medicaid to obtain needed physician services because of their very low reimbursement rates (81).

Most publicly insured adolescents are covered through Medicaid; relatively few are covered through Medicare or CHAMPUS. Medicare coverage is extended only to adolescents with end-stage renal disease, and CHAMPUS coverage is available to adolescents whose parents receive benefits from military service.

Characteristics of Adolescents With Public Health Insurance

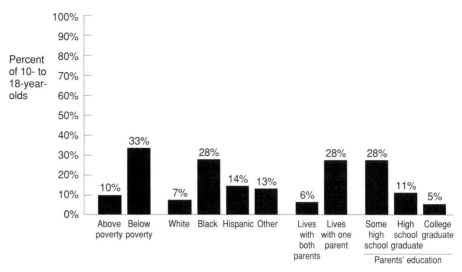

Source: Newacheck, P. W., & McManus, M. A. (1991). Original tabulations from the 1986 National Health Interview Survey.

AMA Profiles of Adolescent Health

Public Insurance

Nine percent of adolescents are covered by public health insurance, primarily Medicaid. The characteristics of publicly insured adolescents appear in the graph:

- Adolescents living in poverty are 3.4 times more likely to have public insurance than those living above the poverty level. However, only one third of all poor adolescents are covered by public health insurance (103). Reasons for this are discussed later in this chapter.

- Black adolescents are 4 times and Hispanics 2 times more likely to have public insurance than white adolescents (103).

- Adolescents living with one parent are 4.7 times more likely to have public insurance than adolescents living with both parents (103).

- Adolescents whose parents have not completed high school are 2.5 times more likely to have public insurance than those whose parents graduated from high school. Adolescents whose parents graduated from high school are twice as likely to have public insurance as those whose parents graduated from college (103).

Regional differences in public coverage of adolescents are minimal. Ten percent of adolescents in the Northeast have public insurance, as do 11% in the Midwest and South and 12% in the West. However, adolescents living in the central city are more than twice as likely as suburban and 1.6 times more likely than rural adolescents to have some form of public coverage (103).

Private health insurance for adolescents

Most adolescents are insured as dependents under a parent's employer-sponsored group health insurance plan. The three major types of such private health insurance plans are (1) traditional plans offered by commercial carriers, (2) health maintenance organizations (HMOs), and (3) preferred provider organizations (PPOs).

Traditional plan: Enrollees select their own physician, and the insurer typically pays a portion of the bill, called a copayment, after a deductible has been met. For example, an insurance company may pay 75% of a medical charge once the individual has paid an annual deductible of, for example, $500. Most group plans place an annual cap on family out-of-pocket expenses (e.g., $2,500), after which insurance pays the full cost of care up to a lifetime maximum benefit level specified in the plan (e.g., $1 million). In efforts to save on expenses, many companies have reduced the value of their health care benefit package by requiring employees to assume greater copayments for health services.

A small proportion of families with adolescents are covered by individual or nongroup plans. Individual and nongroup plans are usually more expensive than group plans, offer less comprehensive benefits, and typically impose exclusions for preexisting conditions.

Health maintenance organizations: Families enrolled in HMOs are generally required to get medical care from physicians who work for the HMO. Ambulatory services are usually provided in the HMO clinic. Local hospitals are contracted to provide reduced rates for inpatient services. Deductibles and cost-sharing requirements are usually minimal, with certain exceptions, such as mental health and substance abuse services.

Preferred provider organizations: PPOs are groups of physicians and hospitals that contract with insurers or employers to provide care at discounted rates. If a family uses a PPO-member physician, the services are usually fully covered, and they pay only the deductible. However, if a non-PPO physician is used, the family may be required to pay a portion of the cost, usually 20% to 30%.

Characteristics of Adolescents With Private Health Insurance

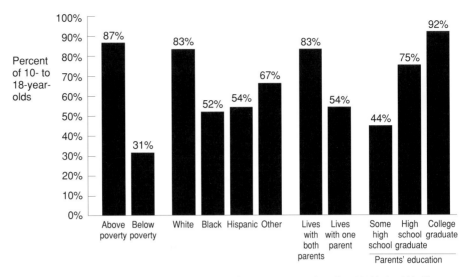

Source: Newacheck, P. W., & McManus, M. A. (1991). Original tabulations from the 1986 National Health Interview Survey.

AMA Profiles of Adolescent Health

Private Insurance

Coverage for privately insured adolescents varies significantly. As shown in the graph:

- Adolescents living above the poverty level are nearly 3 times more likely than adolescents living below the poverty level to have private insurance (103).

- White adolescents are 1.6 times more likely than blacks and 1.5 times more likely than Hispanics to have private health insurance (103).

- Adolescents living with both parents are 1.5 times more likely than adolescents living with one parent to have private health insurance (103).

- Adolescents living with a parent who graduated from college are 1.2 times more likely than those whose parents graduated from high school to have private health insurance, and more than twice as likely as those whose parents did not complete high school (103).

Eighty-one percent of adolescents living in the Northeast and Midwest have private health insurance compared to 70% of adolescents living in the West and South (103).

Suburban adolescents are much more likely to be privately insured than are those living in a rural area or in the central city (82%, 73%, and 64%, respectively) (103).

Changes in Insurance Status Over Time

Most adolescents depend on their parents for insurance. Changes in the economy, parental employment status, and public policy have had a major impact on the number of adolescents covered by health insurance. As of 1986, 64% of uninsured adolescents lived with parents who were uninsured and 41% lived in poor families (71).

The number of uninsured adolescents grew from 3.5 million in 1979 to 4.6 million in 1986, a 1.1 million (25%) increase (71). The major reasons for the growth in the number of uninsured adolescents are as follows:

- The economy is moving away from industrial and manufacturing jobs with generous benefits toward service-sector jobs with few or no health benefits (71).

- As the cost of health insurance increased, many people were unable to meet copayment demands or contribute to private health insurance for themselves or their dependents. The decline in private coverage was much greater among lower-income than middle- and upper-income families (71).

- Between 1979 and 1986, the proportion of privately insured adolescents living in poor families declined by 35%. In contrast, adolescents in middle- and upper-income families declined by less than 2% (71).

- The proportion of adolescents living in poverty increased from 15% in 1979 to 19% in 1986. Although this should have led to

an increase in the proportion covered by Medicaid, greater restrictions in Medicaid eligibility rules resulted in an overall decline in the proportion of poor and near-poor adolescents covered by Medicaid (71).

- The proportion of uninsured adolescents not living with their parents increased substantially, from 61% in 1979 to 74% in 1986. The proportion of adolescents who obtained health insurance benefits from their own jobs declined substantially during this time (71).

Why Adolescents Lack Health Insurance

■ When asked to report why their adolescents have no health insurance coverage, the vast majority of families (72%) cite cost as the major reason (103). As shown in the chart on page 35, other reasons for lack of coverage are:

- parental job layoff or unemployment (13%);

- in good health or does not need insurance (5%);

- unable to obtain insurance because of poor health, illness, or age (1%);

- all other reasons (9%).

Adolescents who work are usually employed in service-industry jobs that do not provide health insurance benefits.

As stated in the previous section, one third of adolescents who live in poverty do not have Medicaid coverage, primarily because the cash assistance level for public assis-

Parents' Reasons Why Their Adolescents Lack Insurance

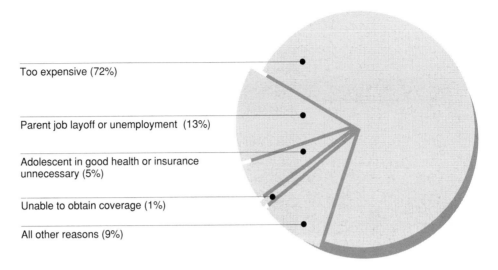

Too expensive (72%)

Parent job layoff or unemployment (13%)

Adolescent in good health or insurance unnecessary (5%)

Unable to obtain coverage (1%)

All other reasons (9%)

Source: Newacheck, P. W., & McManus, M. A. (1991). Original tabulations from the 1986 National Health Interview Survey.

AMA Profiles of Adolescent Health

tance programs is generally set well below the poverty level.

In 1990, President Bush signed into law legislation that will gradually separate Medicaid eligibility from public assistance eligibility. This will eventually allow increased numbers of adolescents from low-income families to gain coverage under the Medicaid program. In the interim, restrictive eligibility standards for Medicaid that exclude the "working poor" continue to account

for the large number of poor adolescents without public insurance. Adolescents whose family income is just above the poverty level are more at risk for being uninsured than adolescents living below the poverty level because they are neither poor enough to qualify for Medicaid nor able to afford private health insurance (103). Recommendations to make insurance more affordable for adolescents and their families are described in chapter 4.

2. What types of adolescent health services are typically covered by private and public health insurance?

Although most adolescents have some form of health insurance, both private and public insurance restricts the amount, scope, and duration of benefits covered. These restrictions may come in the form of exclusions of preexisting conditions, day or dollar limits, restricted

use of providers, prior authorization requirements, low reimbursement, and high cost-sharing requirements. This section summarizes major benefit restrictions used by private insurers and Medicaid.

Private Insurance

Adolescents covered by private health insurance tend to have a full scope of benefits for treatment services such as hospital care, emergency room, acute care office services, and prescription medications (47).

Privately insured adolescents are generally not well insured for such services as preventive care, dental care, outpatient psychiatric treatment, and maternity-related services for dependents. Case management (a benefit offered by a growing number of private and public plans that involves coordinating care for persons who need costly or multiple health services) and individualized benefits management (a flexible benefit arrangement in which benefits such as home care are used in lieu of more expensive benefits such as hospital care) are not well covered (47).

Although most private plans cover mental health and substance abuse services, day limits for both inpatient and outpatient services as well as relatively high cost-sharing requirements are typically imposed to reduce use (47). For example, while many private plans pay 75% to 80% for hospital services, they may reimburse only 50% of outpatient mental health services, up to a maximum dollar amount. Families must then pay the remaining costs.

Private plans generally restrict the settings in which medical care can be provided to hospitals, physicians' offices, and, in some cases, homes, thereby excluding the use of alternative settings such as residential treatment facilities and school-based clinics (47).

Public Insurance

Adolescents with Medicaid are generally well covered for traditional medical services and preventive care. They are less well covered for psychiatric services, physical, occupational, and speech therapy, home health services, substance abuse treatment, case management or care coordination, and nonphysician services provided by psychologists, social workers, and others (48).

Under the Omnibus Budget Reconciliation Act of 1989, new opportunities exist under the Early and

---

The Early and Periodic Screening, Diagnosis, and Treatment Program

The Early and Periodic Screening, Diagnosis, and Treatment (EPSDT) Program ensures that children and adolescents who are eligible for Medicaid are also covered for preventive care. The EPSDT Program provides a comprehensive and periodic assessment of overall health, developmental, and nutritional status and treatment of conditions detected during assessment. It includes vision, dental, and hearing services. The federal government requires that all state Medicaid programs offer EPSDT services to Medicaid-eligible children and adolescents. States are required to establish periodicity schedules for screenings that are based on accepted norms for supervisory care. More frequent screenings are to be provided where medically necessary.

Under the provisions of the Omnibus Budget Reconciliation Act of 1989, the role of the EPSDT Program was greatly expanded. First, providers other than physicians (psychologists, optometrists, nurse practitioners, and some educators) can now provide partial screenings. Second, states must provide any federally authorized Medicaid service that is deemed medically necessary as the result of an EPSDT screen. For example, if a physician determines during an EPSDT screen that speech therapy is medically necessary for an adolescent, the state would be required to provide that service even if it were not usually provided under the state's Medicaid program. This legislation could have profound effects in all states, especially those offering a limited number of services under their Medicaid program.

Periodic Screening, Diagnosis, and Treatment (EPSDT) Program for states to lift the limits on existing benefits and to cover adolescents for additional screening and preventive services (46).

Medical providers have criticized Medicaid for its low reimbursement rates. In a 1989 survey of state Medicaid programs, selected reimbursement rates for routine evaluation and management averaged less than two thirds of private market rates (81).

As a result of low Medicaid reimbursement rates and delays in payment, fewer physicians are participating in Medicaid. For example, between 1978 and 1989, basic participation in the Medicaid program by pediatricians declined from 85% to 77% (137).

3. How well does health insurance protect adolescents and their families from both routine and catastrophic expenses?

Most of the medical services adolescents use are for preventive care and episodic care of acute physical or mental disorders. Because adolescents are rarely hospitalized and tend to use relatively inexpensive ambulatory services, average yearly health expenditures for adolescents are less than half the amount spent on adults of working age and less than one-fifth the amount spent on the elderly (134).

Average Medical Expenses for Adolescent Care

In 1990, the average annual charge for the medical care of an adolescent between 10 and 18 years of age was $612. However, this underestimates the total cost of health care, partly because of the underreporting of medical care for sensitive issues such as substance abuse, mental health problems, and family planning (101).

Substantial variation in medical charges exists between younger and older adolescents. The average total annual charges for medical services to 15- to 18- year-olds ($839) are more than twice those for 10- to 14-year olds ($407) (101). This is largely because older adolescents are more likely to be hospitalized.

Major racial differences in medical charges also exist. White adolescents have average annual charges of $667, twice the $336 annual charges for nonwhites (101). The reason for race differences in medical expenses is not clear but is probably related to the greater hospitalization rate of white adolescents, their greater use of preventive services, or both. This finding warrants further examination.

Gender differences in medical charges are less pronounced. Charges for medical care average $561 a year for adolescent males and $663 for adolescent females, an 18% difference (101). Higher charges for reproductive health services provided to females may contribute to the overall difference.

Adolescents living in poor families tend to have more illnesses and therefore accrue medical charges that are 57% higher than those of adolescents with family incomes

Data on adolescent health care charges and expenses

National data on the use and financial costs of medical services come from three periodic health surveys, the National Medical Care Expenditure Survey (NMCES) conducted in 1977, the National Medical Care Utilization and Expenditure Survey (NMCUES) conducted in 1980, and the National Medical Expenditure Survey (NMES) conducted in 1987. Because data from the NMES are not yet available, most of the data on medical expenses in this chapter are based on the 1980 NMCUES. In NMCUES, one adult in the household reported all medical charges and family expenses for hospital inpatient and outpatient services, physician and nonphysician services, prescribed medications, diagnostic tests, and certain types of medical equipment and supplies, including eyeglasses and contact lenses. Out-of-pocket expenses were defined as the amount of total medical charges paid directly by the family. All financial data, including out-of-pocket expenses, have been converted to 1990 dollars by means of the medical care component of the Consumer Price Index. Information regarding institutional care and certain types of medical supplies and equipment was not collected.

The NMCUES data have two limitations. First, stigmatizing services such as mental health counseling may be underreported. In addition, parents may be unaware of their adolescent's use of certain confidential services, such as family planning.

Second, patterns of health care use and insurance benefits have changed since 1980. Hospital use by adolescents has declined significantly (70) and has been replaced by a wide range of outpatient services (109). Out-of-pocket expenses for many health services, including hospitalization, have increased (49). Insurance premiums have risen dramatically (39), and coverage of selected preventive services and home health care benefits have also increased (49). Changes in medical technology and patterns of care have increased medical expenses in some areas while decreasing expenses in others (109).

Despite these limitations, the NMCUES remains the most current national information base on health care expenditures and sources of payment for adolescents. More recent data will be available when the 1987 NMES is released sometime in 1991 or 1992.

The Adolescent Health Dollar

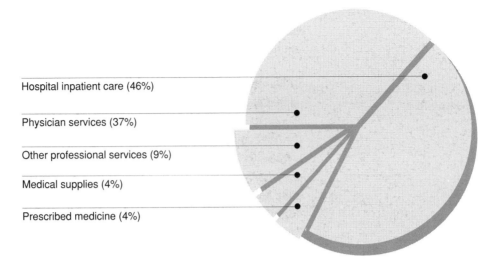

Hospital inpatient care (46%)

Physician services (37%)

Other professional services (9%)

Medical supplies (4%)

Prescribed medicine (4%)

Source: Adapted from Newacheck, P. W., & McManus, M. A. (1990). Health care expenditure patterns for adolescents. *Journal of Adolescent Health Care, 11,* 133-140.

AMA Profiles of Adolescent Health

above the poverty level ($896 and $572, respectively) (101).

▀ Health expenses for adolescents are divided among a number of services. A breakdown of money spent on different types of adolescent health care services appears in the chart:

- The single largest component (46%) of health care expenses for adolescents is inpatient hospital care (101).

- The second leading component of expenses is for physician services (both inpatient and outpatient care), which accounts for more than one third of adolescent health care expenses (101).

- Services provided by nurses, psychologists, physical therapists, and other health professionals account for 9% of adolescent health care expenses (101).

- Medical supplies, prescribed medicine, and other items account for the remaining 8% of adolescent health expenses (101).

Family Out-of-Pocket Spending on Adolescent Medical Care

In most families, out-of-pocket expenses for adolescent health care are low. In 1990, the average cost was $176 for each adolescent. On the average, this represents 29% of the family's total out-of-pocket health care expenses (101).

In 1990, as many as half of all adolescents (17.6 million) had medical expenses below $40, and one third (12.6 million) had no out-of-pocket medical expenses during the course of a year (101).

Adolescents who have no out-of-pocket medical expenses include those who did not use health care services during the year, those who are covered by Medicaid, and those whose families have health insurance with no copayment requirements (101).

Differences in the out-of-pocket share of medical bills families pay for reflect, in part, the nature of health insurance. Historically, private health insurance has offered generous benefits for acute care and hospital services and less generous coverage for outpatient diagnostic and preventive services. This system created financial incentives to use costly inpatient services at times when outpatient settings might have been adequate (101).

- The average medical expenses that families pay depend in part on the type of service received. The share of bills paid directly by a family ranges from an average of 15% for inpatient hospital services to 74% for medical supplies (101).

- On the average, families are required to pay out of pocket 34% of the physician's total charge, 38% of charges by other health professionals, and 70% of charges for prescribed medications. The remaining medical charges are generally paid for by private health insurance, Medicaid, and other third-party payers (101).

Adolescents With High Health Care Expenses

While health care expenses are low for most adolescents, they can be high for adolescents with severe health problems, often causing severe financial strain on the family. Adolescent medical expenses may

also become problematic if the costs of care exceed what adolescents and their families can afford to pay out of pocket for routine care or for more specialized services, such as mental health, alcohol and substance abuse, and reproductive health care. Most families with adolescents have health insurance coverage that offers some protection from burdensome expenses. How well their insurance protects them against a financial catastrophe depends, in part, on whether the adolescent is covered by private or public insurance.

Privately insured families pay an average of 32% of their adolescents' health care bills out of pocket compared to 15% for families with adolescents covered by public health insurance. The higher share of expense paid out of pocket by privately insured families is due, in part, to higher deductibles and coinsurance rates on covered services, as well as to limits on the type and duration of certain services that are typically covered by public insurance plans (101).

Families of adolescents with public insurance coverage pay a lower share of total expenses because their coverage, primarily through Medicaid, requires no cost sharing. Moreover, most poor families covered by Medicaid have few or no discretionary dollars to pay for medical care (101).

Families who are protected least against high medical expenses are, of course, the uninsured. These families pay 62% of their adolescent's medical expenses out of pocket. The remaining expenses are met by charity or result in bad debts (101).

A minority of 10- to 18-year-olds account for the majority of the out-of-pocket adolescent medical care expenses. The 10% of adolescents whose families have the highest out-of-pocket expenses pay more than $350 annually. The amount paid by this group accounts for 65% of all out-of-pocket expenses for adolescents (101).

Pregnancy-related services and childbirth probably account for much of the high medical expenses in the adolescent population. Fifty percent of adolescents are female,

Medical expenses of disabled and nondisabled youth

Direct costs for hospitalization and outpatient care of disabled children and adolescents were estimated in 1980 at $2.9 billion. Missed work by a parent as well as other indirect costs of illness are not included in these estimates. Private insurance and state and federal Programs for Children With Special Health Care Needs, Medicaid, the Supplemental Security Income Disabled Children's Program, the Education for All Handicapped Children's Act, and others help alleviate some family financial burdens but do not cover all of these costs (117).

and they comprise 60% of those with high out-of-pocket expenses. Fifty-eight percent of adolescents with high medical expenses are between the ages of 15 and 18 years (101).

Adolescents most at risk for catastrophic health care expenses are:

- adolescents with a chronic condition or who experience significant physical, psychiatric, or developmental problems. These youth often require a greater amount,

duration, and scope of services than are typically covered by most private and public plans (see chapter 2);

- adolescents insured by plans that do not cover, or impose significant cost-sharing requirements on, a wide array of preventive, primary, and long-term care services, and/or who have insurance plans with high annual out-of-pocket protection and low lifetime limits;

- adolescents living in a poor or near-poor family or who may have other chronically ill family members. These families generally have few discretionary dollars to spend on health care services.

Expenses for Adolescent Mental Health and Substance Abuse Treatment

In 1986, the nation spent approximately $3.5 billion to treat adolescents in special mental health facilities. Nearly half of this money was spent on inpatient care and almost 30% for residential treatment centers. By comparison, outpatient and partial hospitalization services accounted for only about 25% of total expenditures, though they served more than 70% of adolescents receiving mental health care (29).

Adolescents account for a greater share of outpatient mental health care costs than all other age groups combined (25% vs 18%, respectively) and a greater proportion of private psychiatric hospital costs (34% vs 12%, respectively) (124).

In 1987, the mean length of stay in a psychiatric hospital for adolescents was 44 days. At an average cost of $377 a day, each adolescent psychiatric inpatient episode is estimated to be $16,500 (124).

Approximately $185 million was spent in 1987 on adolescent alcohol and drug treatment services—$65 million on alcohol treatment and $120 million on drug treatment (105).

Managed care systems, including health maintenance organizations (HMOs) and preferred provider organizations (PPOs), have expanded during the past several years. These systems were designed to control rising health care costs. However, providers and patients have expressed growing concern that in some cases—particularly those involving mental health and substance abuse treatment—market-driven forces have inappropriately affected medical decision making such that decisions about the nature and extent of care provided do not necessarily coincide with the best interest of the patient.

Expenses for Adolescent Reproductive Health

In 1988, U.S. taxpayers spent nearly $20 billion to support families that began with a birth to an adolescent mother. These costs include Aid to Families With Dependent Children (AFDC), Medicaid, and Food Stamps, but exclude other public costs typically associated with family support, such as housing subsidies, special education, foster care, and day care.

In 1988, there were 488,941 births to women under the age of 20 years. Of these, 45,664 (9%) were low-birth-weight infants (90). Based on average hospital costs of between $11,670 and $39,420 per low-birth-weight infant (125), the hospital costs for low-birth-weight infants of adolescent mothers ranged from $533 million to $1.8 billion.

The Center for Population Options estimates that if every birth to an adolescent mother had been delayed, the U.S. would have saved $8 billion (120). For every dollar spent on quality prenatal care, more than $3 can be saved by reducing the number of low-birth-weight babies (131).

Health care expenses for adolescents vary enormously. Out-of-pocket expenses are low for most families because adolescents use relatively few health services. For these adolescents, insurance generally provides adequate protection against undue financial hardship. Out-of-pocket costs are greatest among adolescents whose families are uninsured or underinsured, adolescents who use pregnancy-related services, and those who are disabled or chronically ill. Expanded opportunities to obtain quality health care coverage, as outlined in chapter 4, would greatly benefit these families.

4. What are the consequences of being uninsured?

Given the complicated nature of many adolescent health problems and the fact that 4.7 million adolescents have neither public nor private insurance, it is important to examine the consequences of being uninsured. Little research on access to care, however, has linked health insurance coverage with health status. Most research has focused on the relationship between insurance coverage and use of health services.

Uninsured adolescents have fewer physician services and wait longer between visits. Adolescents with health insurance are 1.3 times more likely than those who are uninsured to have visited a physician for routine medical care within the past year (29).

Hospitalization rates for adolescents are similar regardless of health insurance status. Eighteen percent of adolescent hospital episodes were for uninsured youth (103).

Only 70% of uninsured 12- to 17-year-olds have a regular source of care, compared to 90% of insured adolescents (29).

Adolescents most in need of coverage—those in fair or poor health—are twice as likely to be uninsured and 3 times more likely to be publicly insured than adolescents in excellent health (102).

Because of preexisting conditions, uninsured disabled youth often have difficulty obtaining private insurance coverage. Unless they qualify for Medicaid or a state health insurance plan, including high-risk pools and catastrophic plans, uninsured disabled youth are likely to become medically uninsurable.

Summary and Implications

The availability and quality of health insurance have a major impact on the medical care that adolescents receive. In the current health care financing system, most adolescents from middle- and upper-income families are privately insured through their parents' employer-based plans. Adolescents from poor families are more likely to be publicly insured, primarily through Medicaid. During the last decade there has been a dramatic erosion in health insurance coverage for adolescents in the United States, leaving almost 5 million 10- to 18-year-olds without coverage. Uninsured adolescents are concentrated among the poor and near poor, minorities (particularly Hispanics), and those in fair or poor health. The 15% of adolescents who fall through the cracks of the U.S. health care financing system are often ineligible for public insurance or live in families that cannot afford or are ineligible for private health insurance. Without health insurance, adolescents are far more likely to delay seeking medical attention for preventive and primary care.

Even among insured families, the quality of coverage is often inconsistent, with inadequate coverage for preventive care and specialized services, such as mental health, substance abuse, rehabilitative, or dental care (47). Thus, even insured adolescents face significant barriers to obtaining needed services.

From this review, it is also clear that health insurance does not provide the scope and breadth of services needed to prevent and treat many of the health problems experienced by today's adolescents. Although insurance was originally developed to provide coverage for major medical expenses, adolescents are in great need of coverage that emphasizes prevention and that more adequately addresses the complex problems of today's youth.

Chapter

3.

What are the nonfinancial barriers to health services for adolescents?

Even if all adolescents were adequately covered by health insurance, many would still not receive the services they need. The reasons for this are complex but can be divided into two basic areas, one reflecting the organization of the health care system and the other related to the psychosocial development of adolescents.

This chapter examines nonfinancial barriers to care, including fragmentation and lack of coordination among health care providers, issues of patient-provider confidentiality, the training of health providers in adolescent health care, features of clinical practice, and fears and concerns that deter some adolescents from seeking care.

The questions addressed in this section are:

1. **In what ways does the organization of health care services limit health care use by adolescents?**

2. **What other factors impede adolescents' use of health services?**

1. In what ways does the organization of health care services limit health care use by adolescents?

Obtaining appropriate health services can be difficult for any adolescent, but it is especially difficult for those who are uninsured or underinsured, have multiple health problems, or live in medically underserved areas. Many features of the medical system limit the use of health services by adolescents. These include an insufficient number and maldistribution of primary care physicians as well as public and community programs. The fragmentation and lack of coordinated health services, inadequate training for physicians and health providers in adolescent health, and features of office practice also pose barriers to adolescents' use of health services. A lack of sensitivity by physicians and health providers to developmental issues and cultural background of adolescents, and adolescents' concerns about whether information shared during the medical visit will remain confidential, also deter some adolescents from seeking necessary health care.

Availability of Physicians and Public Health Programs

The American health care system has been described as a two-tiered system in which families and adolescents with private health insurance coverage receive care from private physicians, while the uninsured and those with public insurance receive care from public or community programs.

In 1988, 83% of 12- to 17-year-olds saw a physician for routine health care. However, only 54% of central-city adolescents and 50% of rural adolescents visited a doctor for routine health care. This is partly because fewer physicians practice in these areas (29).

The number of practicing primary care physicians has declined dramatically over the past several decades. During the 1930s, 80% of practicing physicians were in primary care compared to fewer than 25% today (4).

The overall proportion of nonfederal, patient-care physicians working in rural areas fell from 15% in 1970 to 12% in 1986, due mostly to a decline in general practitioners (13).

The availability of community health services provided to mostly low-income adolescents is left to the discretion of state and local governments. Block grants, through Title V state Maternal and Child Health programs, provide limited funding for direct service programs, including specialty clinics for pregnant and parenting adolescents, comprehensive evaluation programs for adolescents with developmental disorders, and nutritional services.

- The purpose of Maternal and Child Health block grants to states is to (a) assure access to quality maternal and child health services for those with low incomes and those who live in areas with limited available health services, (b) increase the number of children and adolescents living in low-income families who receive health assessments and follow-up diagnostic and treatment services, (c) promote the health of mothers and children, and (d) encourage collaboration and coordination with other federal programs to promote health and increase access.

Fragmentation and Lack of Coordinated Care

In addition to primary and preventive medical care, many adolescents need additional health-related services. Such services include nutritional assessment and counseling, mental health and substance abuse counseling, family assessment and counseling, and school and community disease prevention and health promotion programs.

For the individual physician or health professional, coordination of care means arranging or offering in the office a range of health services, as well as knowing about existing community services to which adolescents can be referred. For the community at large, coordination means ensuring that agencies collaborate to make sure that adolescents receive needed health services.

Most health services supported by public funds are organized categorically, for example, by pregnancy, child abuse, substance abuse, or mental health. However, a young person in need of one type of service frequently needs others as well. The categorical nature of health services can be detrimental to adolescents with multiple problems that require extensive and coordinated care (93).

Increasingly, state lawmakers are developing public policy to facilitate the interagency coordination of services. Flexible funding strategies, interagency case management, local councils to coordinate services, and family-oriented policies are recent legislative innovations (see chapter 4).

Professional Training in Adolescent Health

Many health professionals report that their professional training did not provide them with the skills needed to manage the complex social and emotional problems of adolescents effectively. As a result, many are unable to recognize, diagnose, or properly treat adolescents with complex health problems.

Availability of physicians with specialty training in adolescent care

Approximately 1,000 physicians list adolescent medicine as a specialty interest in the AMA master file of all physicians in the United States. Most of these physicians are trained in pediatrics, general and family practice, internal medicine, or psychiatry. Currently, there is one adolescent medicine specialist for every 20,500 adolescents and one child and adolescent psychiatrist for every 5,000 adolescents (54).

The Maternal and Child Health Bureau of the Department of Health and Human Services funds six interdisciplinary training programs in adolescent health. Trainees include adolescent medicine physicians as well as graduate students in nutrition, psychology, nursing, and social work. Since the inception of these programs in 1977, almost 700 professionals have been trained in them, 23% from medicine, 15% from nursing, 14% from nutrition, 30% from psychology, and 18% from social work (23).

Currently, 39 adolescent medicine fellowship programs graduate around 60 physicians each year. Most offer 1 to 2 years of specialty training to pediatricians, internists, and family physicians. All programs are sponsored by departments of pediatrics or children's hospitals (63). Additional information about professional training in adolescent health care appears in chapters 3 and 4.

Health Professionals' Assessment of Their Training in Adolescent Health

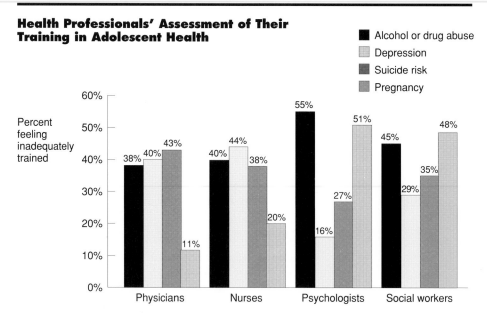

Legend:
- Alcohol or drug abuse
- Depression
- Suicide risk
- Pregnancy

Percent feeling inadequately trained

Physicians: 38%, 40%, 43%, 11%
Nurses: 40%, 44%, 38%, 20%
Psychologists: 55%, 16%, 27%, 51%
Social workers: 45%, 29%, 35%, 48%

Source: Blum, R. W., & Bearinger, L. H. (1990). Knowledge and attitudes of health professionals toward adolescent health care. *Journal of Adolescent Health Care, 11,* 289-294.

AMA Profiles of Adolescent Health

Fifty percent of primary care physicians nationwide reported insufficient training related to psychosocial, behavioral, and mental health problems (30). Not surprisingly, psychiatrists felt significantly more competent than physicians in other specialties to manage these adolescent health problems (108).

■ Primary care physicians, nurses, psychologists, and social workers who participated in a national survey were asked to rate their skills in 16 different problem areas (31). As shown in the graph:

• Nearly 40% of physicians and nurses believe they are unprepared to treat adolescents who have alcohol or drug abuse problems, who are depressed, or who are at risk for suicide. A much smaller proportion (11% and 20%, respectively) thought they were insufficiently trained to manage adolescent pregnancy (31).

• Nearly 40% of psychologists and social workers report insufficient training in managing adolescent alcohol or drug abuse problems or adolescent pregnancy. Most felt better trained to manage depression (31).

Intensive training can substantially improve professional skills and attitudes toward adolescents. A study of pediatric residents in Los Angeles found that those who completed an intensive rotation in adolescent medicine showed significant improvement in their clinical skills, comfort in dealing with adolescents, and appreciation of adolescents when compared to those who did not complete the rotation (98).

A study of Midwestern pediatricians, family physicians, internists, and obstetricians-gynecologists found that relatively few had comprehensive training in adolescent medicine. Seven percent reported having had no training in adolescent medicine. Of those who did receive training, 39% were trained during their residency and 45% through continuing education courses after their residency. Only 15% received training in adolescent medicine both during and after residency (108).

Physicians generally receive little formal education in the prevention or treatment of alcohol or other drug abuse. A survey of U.S. pediatric training programs found that only 44% of medical student programs and 40% of residency training programs require formal instruction in these areas. Few offered an elective course in alcohol or substance abuse for medical students or residents (27% and 34%, respectively). Curriculum time constraints, the lack of a qualified instructor, and the lack of funds to care for these patients were found seriously to impede formal training in the prevention and treatment of alcohol and drug abuse (2).

A major barrier to the incorporation of prevention in primary care is the lack of agreement among medical organizations, federal agencies, and advisory groups about the content and periodicity of preventive health examinations. The major differences surround whether most adolescents should be examined once per year or every other year. Opinions also differ about the type of screening that should be used.

Guidelines developed for the average adolescent may fail to take into account needs of youth with special needs, those who are poor, or those whose parents are not competent caretakers.

Although various groups of health professionals should develop and incorporate material about adolescents into training and continuing education programs, interest in these opportunities by health professionals appears to be limited. Only 32% of physicians, 40% of psychologists, and 49% of social workers expressed interest in developing skills tailored to the health concerns of adolescents (31).

Time Demands

Time restraints in busy private practice settings can make it difficult to provide adolescents an appropriate level of health care. In one study, 37% of physicians and nurses, 33% of social workers, and 46% of psychologists viewed time demands as a major barrier to treating adolescents (31). However, time is a critical part of building rapport. Better rapport may encourage the adolescents to ask questions or mention problems to health professionals that might not otherwise be raised.

Under current practice conditions, the average office visit does not allow enough time for physicians to screen thoroughly for all important physical and psychosocial problems an adolescent may be experiencing. Many adolescents contact physicians because of complaints that turn out to be symptoms of more complex psychosocial problems that may require more lengthy counseling, assessment, or referral.

It is estimated that a complete history and physical examination for a new adolescent patient take approximately 30 to 45 minutes and somewhat less time for an adolescent receiving ongoing care (79).

Nearly half of adolescent visits with office-based physicians last 10 minutes or less, 30% last 11 to 15 minutes, and 22% last 16 minutes or more (99). Visits generally last longer in school-based health centers, where only 19% of visits last less than 10 minutes, 35% last 10 to 20 minutes, and 45% last more than 20 minutes (73).

Sensitivity of Health Professionals

Potential pitfalls in the health professional's attitude toward the adolescent include stereotyping of the adolescent as a "problem," the desire to avoid becoming involved in problem areas having to do with sex or substance use, and underestimating the complexity of the social and mental health issues affecting the adolescent (118).

It is important that physicians and other health professionals develop skills for communicating with adolescents whose racial, ethnic, religious, or economic background differs from their own. Health professionals who lack an understanding or sensitivity to cultural issues facing an adolescent may have difficulty obtaining accurate health information, fail to identify an adolescent at risk for violence, injury, or suicide, or inadvertently increase anxiety about the visit (45).

For example, it might be useful for health professionals to know that in many Southeast Asian cultures, a clan leader other than the parent sometimes controls medical treatment. Thus, it is important for the health professional to identify the primary authority figure in the family if full cooperation with medical procedures is to be realized (104).

Recognition of a family's non-Western medical practices may enhance compliance with a treatment protocol (104).

Barriers to care for disabled adolescents

There are an estimated 2 million adolescents with chronic illnesses (100). Adolescents with disabilities have special health needs that require coordinated services, especially as they make the transition from pediatric to adult medical care. Former Surgeon General C. Everett Koop, M.D., noted that adolescents with disabilities who have come to rely on pediatric health services may be reluctant to change to the adult health care system, viewing it as less supportive and coordinated (91).

Several barriers have been identified that affect the medical care of disabled adolescents: (1) limited physician knowledge of many disabling conditions; (2) limited physician knowledge of available community resources; (3) limited physician training in adolescent development regardless of the presence of a disabling condition; (4) reluctance by some pediatricians to turn over medical care to an internist because of their deep familiarity with the patient and uncertainty that another physician could provide the same level of care; and (5) reluctance by internists to assume responsibility for conditions with which they have limited familiarity (91).

Parents of chronically ill youth who participated in a national survey conducted by the General Accounting Office recommended improving access to needed services by (1) alleviating financial problems resulting from limitations in health insurance coverage, (2) consolidating information on existing services and making it available to all organizations serving chronically ill children and adolescents, (3) providing this information to parents during the hospital discharge process, and (4) referring parents who need help in the home care setting to organizations providing case management services (130).

More research is needed on communication between adolescents and health providers, to help providers avoid common pitfalls and improve communication and trust. Such research must take into account differences in the gender, racial, ethnic, religious, and economic backgrounds of providers and the adolescent patient.

Office Policies and Medical Settings

Many pediatricians discontinue seeing patients when they enter adolescence despite the 1988 endorsement by the American Academy of Pediatrics to continue pediatric care through age 21 years, and beyond in some instances, for youth with chronic illnesses or disabilities (8).

Since the early 1980s, the proportion of pediatricians treating adolescents has increased. In 1989, 88% of the members of the American Academy of Pediatrics reported that they provide care to adolescents (136).

Office decor and materials in the waiting room that are relevant to adolescents may reduce barriers to care. Baby toys, story books, or magazines geared primarily to adults make many adolescents feel out of place (64). Appropriate reading materials may enhance adolescents' comfort and feeling of being accepted (42).

Scheduling visits at the end of the day when small children are not in the office and the physician has more time available may also enhance the adolescent's feeling of comfort and acceptance.

Confidentiality

Confidentiality is generally acknowledged as essential to maintain a patient's trust and to elicit necessary information (92). However, confidential health services for adolescents are legally available only under specific conditions:

- for the diagnosis and treatment of a sexually transmitted disease;

- for the diagnosis of pregnancy;

- when emergency care is required;

- when a court has given consent for a minor to be treated (the "mature minor" concept);

- when the individual is an "emancipated" minor, that is, an adolescent who is married, who is serving in the armed forces, who lives away from home because the parent is unavailable or may be unwilling or unable to be involved, or who has run away or been forced out of the parent's home (44). In all other situations, parental approval or notification is necessary.

Independent and confidential health care is also important for the adolescent who, though living at home, needs treatment for a problem that he or she is unwilling to reveal to parents. Sexual activity, venereal disease, drug abuse, and mental distress and depression are typical examples. Adolescents whose parents have refused consent or who contribute to a problem (such as sexual abuse) also need independent confidential care (44).

Adolescents' Willingness to Seek Health Care Depending on Parental Involvement

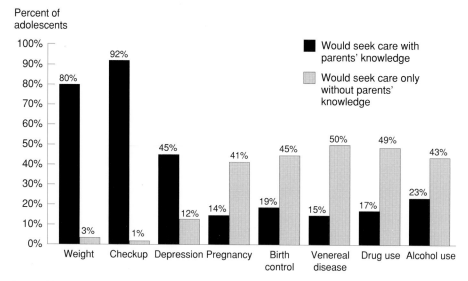

Source: Marks, A., Malizio, J., Hoch, J., Brody, R., & Fisher, M. (1983). Assessment of health needs and willingness to utilize health care resources of adolescents in a surburban population. *Journal of Pediatrics, 102*, 456-460.

AMA Profiles of Adolescent Health

■ Adolescents' belief that physicians will divulge information obtained during an office visit to a parent or legal authority is often cited as a reason why they do not seek needed health services, particularly for sensitive issues. A survey of suburban adolescents found that the nature of the health problem had a strong bearing on the adolescent's desire for confidential health care and whether or not health services were sought. As shown below:

• The vast majority of adolescents are willing to seek routine care with parental knowledge. On the other hand, if parental knowledge were mandatory, only 45% of adolescents would seek health services for depression, and fewer than 20% would seek care related to birth control, venereal disease, or drug use (80).

• Only about two thirds of adolescents report that they are willing to see a physician for important health conditions with or without parental knowledge (80).

Most states require parental consent before general medical care is given to a minor. Parental consent requirements presume that a minor lacks the emotional and intellectual capacity to make important decisions and needs the guidance and protection of a parent. Consent regulations also presume that parents are legally responsible for their adolescent's well-being and will act in their child's best interest, that they should be involved in important services offered to their adolescent, and that they are financially liable for their care (44).

In recent years, some states have replaced the parental consent requirement with a parental notification requirement for health services related to sexual activity, drug and alcohol abuse, and mental health issues. Currently, fewer than one fourth of the states have statutes requiring parental notification for a minor's decision to terminate a pregnancy electively (51).

All states have laws allowing physicians to diagnose and treat adolescents for a sexually transmitted disease without parental consent. The physician's right to prescribe birth control or perform an abortion without parental consent remains a matter of debate at both the national and state levels (60).

Even when state law does not require parental notification or consent, confidential health services may be denied to adolescents by hospitals, clinics, health maintenance organizations, individual physicians, or insurance companies. This policy reflects, in part, health providers' concerns that if a minor does not pay for the services provided, parents may also not pay when they did not consent to the service or were not notified about it (51).

A 1987 national AMA survey found that physicians are more likely than the general public to support confidential health services for adolescents, though their support depends, in part, on the age of the adolescent. Thirty-nine percent of physicians and 30% of the public favor confidential health services for 12- to 14-year-olds. Sixty-three percent of physicians and 50% of the public support confidential health services for 15- to 17-year-olds (56).

Younger physicians and obstetrician-gynecologists are more likely than older physicians and physicians in other medical specialities to express support for the use of confidential health services for adolescents (106).

Most physicians who support confidential care encourage parental involvement when it would benefit the adolescent, but they would not make notification a prerequisite for treatment (75).

In summary, various features of the U.S. health care delivery system pose barriers for an adolescent who might otherwise seek health care. The shift away from primary care to medical subspecialization has reduced continuity of care, which is important for the adolescent. Most physicians receive little training in adolescent health and, therefore, have limited opportunities to develop effective communication and other skills that are developmentally appropriate for adolescents. Time demands clearly place additional constraints on adolescent use of health care services. Finally, patient-provider confidentiality and consent laws deter some adolescents from seeking needed care, and physicians need to address these concerns directly with adolescents and their parents. Policy recommendations by medical societies on confidential health services for adolescents appear in chapter 4.

2. What other factors impede adolescents' use of health services?

Even if all adolescents were covered by health insurance and health services available to them in the community, some adolescents would probably not receive needed health care, for reasons related to psychosocial development, gender, or other characteristics. For example, egocentrism, which normally peaks during early to mid-adolescence, may lead an adolescent to feel invulnerable, exempt from particular illnesses or the consequences of risky behavior (43). This self-conception may also lead an adolescent to ignore, deny, or fail to recognize a medical problem that exists, perhaps hoping that the problem will go away on its own. As a result of the delay in seeking care, a medical condition may deteriorate to the point that more expensive and elaborate medical treatment is required. Fear, embarrassment, denial, and lack of knowledge about health issues also deter some adolescents from seeking needed health services.

Although they are sexually active at younger ages, adolescent males are significantly less likely than adolescent females to discuss contraception with a physician (77).

After the age of 10 years, females are more likely than males to be diagnosed as depressed. It appears, however, that females may internalize problems and tensions, while males may express depression by engaging in risk-taking or acting out. As a result, males may not seek care for the mental and emotional difficulty they may have, instead entering the health care system after a physical injury.

Fear, Embarrassment, and Denial

Real or imagined fears that may deter some adolescents from seeking care include:

- discomfort, pain, or embarrassment associated with the visit (e.g., gynecologic examination) (42);

- fear that the physician may find that "something is really wrong" (42);

- perceived adverse side effects (e.g., from some types of contraceptives) (42);

- concern about reputation if friends or family found out about the visit (112);

- anticipated disapproval by the physician (112);

- lack of confidentiality (112);

- concern that seeking care will create conflict with parents (112).

Topics Adolescents Want to and Actually Discuss With Physicians

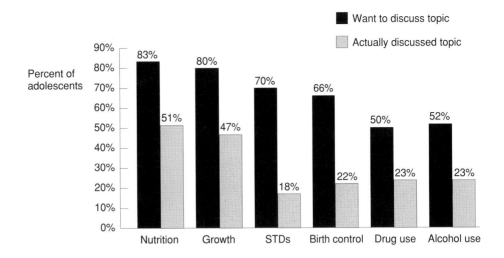

Source: Malus, M., LaChance, P. A., Lamy, L., Macaulay, A., & Vanasse, M. (1987). Priorities in adolescent health care: The teenager's viewpoint. *Journal of Family Practice, 25,* 159-162.

AMA Profiles of Adolescent Health

▰ Among adolescents in general, a gap exists between topics they say they want to discuss with a physician and those they actually talk about when given the opportunity. A survey of adolescents living in Montreal found:

• More than 80% of adolescents said they would like to talk with their physicians about body changes during adolescence, including nutrition, growth, and physical fitness, though only about 50% actually did so when given the opportunity.

• Between 60% and 80% of adolescents said they would like to talk with their physicians about sexually transmitted diseases (STDs) and contraception; half wanted to talk about how reproductive organs work and about secondary sex characteristics, kissing, petting, and intercourse. However, only one third to one half of ado-

lescents actually did so when given the opportunity (77).

• Between 50% and 60% wanted to talk with their physicians about alcohol consumption, drug use, feelings of depression, and lack of confidence, but fewer than 25% actually did so when given the opportunity (77).

There are several reasons why many of these topics are not discussed. Some adolescents are too shy and uncomfortable with their bodies to raise sensitive but important health issues. Some may view the physician as too distant, aloof, rushed, or unwilling to discuss certain topics (77). However, adolescents appear to welcome increased communication with their physicians if made to feel comfortable doing so.

Barriers to Care for Sexually Transmitted Diseases

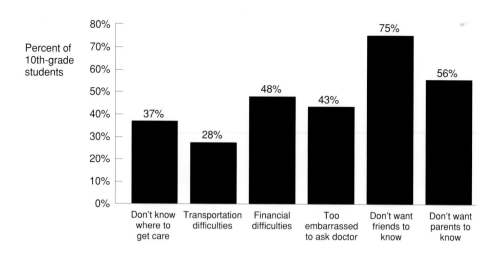

Source: American School Health Association, Association for the Advancement of Health Education, & Society for Public Health Education, Inc. (1989). *The National Adolescent Student Health Survey: A report on the health of America's youth.* Oakland, CA: Third Party Publishing Company.

AMA Profiles of Adolescent Health

A 1987 national survey of 10th graders found that many adolescents do not know where to go for or are too embarrassed to seek medical treatment of sexually transmitted diseases. As shown in the graph:

• Fewer than 40% know where to go for treatment of a sexually transmitted disease, nearly half said that they would have difficulty paying for treatment, and more than one fourth said that transportation would deter them from getting care (22).

• Embarrassment and reputation were also major barriers to care. Forty-three percent said they would be embarrassed to ask a doctor what was wrong if they had a sexually transmitted disease, 75% did not want their friends to know, and 56% did not want their parents to know (22).

An adolescent's denial often hampers the physician's ability to diagnose and treat a problem properly. This is especially difficult among adolescents who abuse substances (68) and those who are pregnant.

Knowledge

Many adolescents receive health and sex education in their school, religious organization, youth group, or family. However, for many the instruction has little impact. Moreover, information alone does not necessarily change behavior.

In a 1986 survey of high school seniors, 72% said that they had a drug education course in school. However, only 39% rated these discussions as being of considerable or great value, and 40% said that the course had not changed their interest in trying drugs (25).

One in four sexually active adolescents will contract a sexually transmitted disease before graduating from high school (116). However, 40% of adolescents are unable to recognize common symptoms of a sexually transmitted disease, and fewer than one third know that public health departments will provide confidential care to adolescents with a sexually transmitted disease (22).

Although the majority of 10th-grade students have not yet had sexual intercourse, most will during the next 2 years (50). To reduce the risks of unprotected sex, adolescents need appropriate information about and access to effective contraception, as well as treatment for sexually transmitted diseases.

It is important to improve comprehensive health education by making it more meaningful for children and adolescents. Health education should help adolescents overcome feelings of fear, embarrassment, and denial and encourage them to contact a physician or other health professional with questions or problems. Adolescents also need instruction on how to use the health care system effectively. While knowledge alone may not translate into healthy behavior, accurate, detailed information about sexual issues, substance use, and other health-threatening behaviors is essential for adolescents to make healthy decisions and avoid unnecessary risk-taking behavior.

Summary and Implications

Characteristics of the health care system and developmental charac-teristics of adolescents pose important nonfinancial barriers to care. Organizational barriers can be reduced as more physicians and health providers are trained and willing to see adolescents, as additional public and community programs are developed to reach adolescents, and as private settings adapt to adolescent needs and interests. To facilitate open communication with providers and encourage appropriate use of health services in a timely fashion, health providers need to discuss confidentiality with the adolescent and his or her family. Most parents understand and accept confidential care for their adolescent once advised of its importance to their adolescent's well-being. Providers who cannot assure confidentiality may choose to refer the adolescent to a community program where confidentiality can be guaranteed.

Some adolescents are better prepared than others to assume responsibility for their own health care. Some find the health care system confusing and overwhelming, are unable to arrange for an appointment on their own, forget to keep an appointment, or are unable to comply with a physician's instructions without adult monitoring. Some cannot recognize symptoms of medical and emotional problems and do not know where to go for help even when aware that a problem exists. With appropriate education at school and at home, these and other barriers to health services can, in large part, be overcome.

4.

What can be done to improve access to health services for adolescents?

Current health care financing in the United States leaves one in seven adolescents without health insurance and many more without coverage for needed services. As shown in earlier chapters, these problems are most acute for adolescents living in poor or near-poor families, for minority youth, and for adolescents with disabilities. Numerous proposals that would better meet the needs of uninsured and underinsured adolescents are currently under discussion by policymakers, legislators, and others. One of the critical issues in public and private initiatives is whether improving health insurance coverage for adolescents should be developed separately from other age groups or combined with initiatives targeting all children and youth or all Americans.

This chapter examines selected policy options for reducing the size of the uninsured adolescent population, specifically Medicaid reforms and the expansion of employer-sponsored private insurance. Selected proposals by organized medicine to improve access are also described. The chapter also examines strategies for reducing high out-of-pocket expenditures for adolescent health care and concludes by offering recommendations that would minimize or eliminate some of the nonfinancial barriers to health care.

The questions addressed in this chapter are:

1. What are the major policy options for reducing the number of uninsured and underinsured adolescents?

2. What other steps could ensure that adolescents receive needed health care services?

1. What are the major policy options for reducing the number of uninsured and underinsured adolescents?

Several proposals that would reform the health care financing system in the United States are currently being considered. Most of them would incorporate mandated employer coverage of employees and dependents and would expand public insurance through Medicaid or other public programs for those without ties to the labor market. This section reviews the effects of these two policy strategies on reducing the number of uninsured adolescents.

Expansion of Medicaid

Currently, each state sets its own financial eligibility thresholds for Medicaid under broad federal guidelines. This has resulted in

Public opinion favors increased spending and services for adolescent health

Children and adolescents constitute about one third of all uninsured Americans. Medicaid, the single largest public funding source for children's and adolescents' health care, currently assists only about one third of all poor adolescents. A 1990 national survey reported that more than 70% of Americans approve of increased spending on children's and adolescents' health care despite the national budget deficit. This sentiment was shared by age, economic, and racial and ethnic groups and by voters in the major political groups (65% of Democrats, 51% of Republicans, and 61% of independent voters). Fifty-nine percent of Americans said that they would accept a tax increase of $100 a year, the cost estimated to provide health insurance to all uninsured children and adolescents (89).

large differences among state eligibility criteria for adolescents.

In 1989, categorical eligibility thresholds for a family of three ranged from as low as $118 per month in Alabama to a high of $846 in Alaska (48). This means, for ex-

ample, that a mother with two adolescent children in Alabama would not be eligible for Medicaid if her income after deductions for child care and work-related expenses exceeded $118 per month.

In 1989, Congress mandated that all states cover pregnant women and children under 6 years of age whose family income is below 133% of the federal poverty level. In 1990, Congress mandated a further phased-in expansion in coverage of 6- to 18-year-olds living in families whose income was below 100% of the federal poverty level. Eligibility for mandated Medicaid coverage, which used to end at a child's 6th birthday, will rise by 1 year annually during the next 13 years (26).

Changes in federal law to establish a uniform national standard for eligibility would greatly reduce or eliminate existing inequities between states. In 1990, the federal poverty level was $10,560 for a family of three.

If a national eligibility cutoff was established immediately at the federal poverty level, an additional 1.9 million uninsured adolescents aged 10 to 18 years would become eligible for Medicaid coverage. This policy alone would reduce the uninsured adolescent population by 37%.

If eligibility were set at 200% of the poverty level, a total of 3.4 million uninsured adolescents would be-

Proposals by organized medicine to improve access to medical care

The AMA, as well as each of the major primary care specialties that treat adolescents, have proposed reforms that would increase access to health services, improve the quality of care, reduce costs, and increase patient and provider satisfaction with the health care system. A brief overview of each proposal appears below.

American Medical Association: The American Medical Association has proposed "Health Access America," a 16-point plan to improve access to affordable, quality health care. The proposal recommends extending access, controlling inappropriate health care cost increases, sustaining the Medicare program, and promoting prevention. The end objective is to ensure that every citizen has access to health insurance and, thus, the benefits of the American health care system. The AMA proposal calls for Medicaid and Medicare reform, employer-mandated coverage for all full-time employees and their families, the creation of state risk pools, expanded private-sector financing for long-term care, reform of professional liability, the development of practice parameters, changes in the tax treatment of employee health care benefits, encouragement of cost-conscious decisions, innovative insurance underwriting, expanded federal support for medical education and research, increased efforts at health promotion and disease prevention by physicians and patients, facilitation of fair competition between self-insured plans and state-regulated health insurance policies, reduced administrative costs of health care delivery, and encouragement of physicians to practice in accordance with the highest ethical standards, with voluntary care for persons without insurance and who cannot afford health insurance. This proposal also includes a standard benefits program. Further information can be obtained by writing "Health Access America," American Medical Association, 515 N. State Street, Chicago, IL 60610.

American Academy of Pediatrics: This proposal would guarantee all children through age 21 years and all pregnant women financial access to necessary, appropriate, and effective health care services, regardless of family income, employment status, ethnic origin, geographic location, or health status. A one-class system of medical care would be established by replacing the portion of the Medicaid program currently serving children and pregnant women with private insurance offering uniform benefits. All segments of society, including individuals, the private sector, and government, would have a shared responsibility for funding the system. The patient would choose an insurance plan and his or her physicians; similarly, physicians would choose acceptable plans and case loads. Compensation for services would be set by the marketplace, not the federal government. Costs would be contained through increased use of preventive services, use of case managers, and cost sharing. Administrative procedures would make this system user friendly. Further information can be obtained by writing to the American Academy of Pediatrics, Department of Government Liaison, 1331 Pennsylvania Avenue N.W., Suite 721N, Washington, DC 20004.

American Academy of Family Physicians: The AAFP supports providing access to the nation's uninsured through a combination of private and public financing mechanisms. The Academy supports employer-mandated coverage for all full-time employees and their families (with the exception of some small employers), cost-sharing requirements between employers and employees with a maximum annual cap on out-of-pocket expenditures, regional risk pools, a basic range of services included in employer-purchased coverage, a substantially revised Medicaid program that includes uniform income-based national eligibility criteria for

come eligible for Medicaid, thus reducing the uninsured adolescent population by 70% (71). Clearly, establishing standard age and income eligibility levels for Medicaid would significantly improve adolescents' access to funding for health care services.

Expansion of Private Health Insurance

Many uninsured adolescents will not benefit from the expansions of Medicaid described above because their family income is too high. For this group, initiatives to expand private health insurance may be more appropriate. Several medical groups

Medicaid, a uniform package of Medicaid benefits consistent with employer-sponsored insurance plans, comparable reimbursement for Medicare and Medicaid services, and Medicaid coverage for low-income individuals and their dependents who are not otherwise covered under an employer-sponsored insurance program. Further information can be obtained by writing the American Academy of Family Physicians, 8880 Ward Parkway, Kansas City, MO 64114.

American College of Physicians: The ACP has proposed comprehensive reform and the establishment of universal access, a system in which coverage is available to everyone regardless of health status and everyone is entitled to the same benefits. Costs could be offset by administrative savings, the reallocation of resources, or some combination of individual and employer premiums and government subsidies as needed. The ACP lists 16 criteria for a better health care system, categorized in terms of benefits, financing, organization and delivery, and satisfaction. The criteria include a mechanism for determining the scope of benefits, uniform benefits for all, coverage decisions based on clinical effectiveness, and continuity of coverage and benefits that are independent of residence or employment. It calls for financing to be adequate to eliminate financial barriers to needed care, mechanisms for controlling costs, minimizing administrative expenses as well as procedures, and professional liability costs, and the incorporation of existing revenue sources into new financing systems. The position paper also calls for an infrastructure to deliver health care services efficiently and effectively, mechanisms to assure quality, innovation, and improvement, a flexible system, and incentives to encourage individuals to take responsibility for their health, seek preventive health care, and pursue health promotion activities. The ACP also urges the development of a system that ensures that patients, physicians, and other health care professionals are satisfied. Further information can be obtained by writing to the American College of Physicians, Independence Mall West, Sixth Street at Race, Philadelphia, PA 19106-1572.

American Society of Internal Medicine: This proposal has four basic components that include the expansion of employer-based health insurance, improvement and expansion of public financing, coverage for long-term care, and reductions in health care costs and other barriers to care. The expansion of employer-based health insurance involves mandated coverage of a basic benefits package with special assistance to small businesses, in the form of regional insurers, risk pools, federal subsidies, tax deductions, and other strategies. It also calls for tax incentives for individuals and for reform in the market for health insurance by prohibiting experience rating and preexisting condition exclusions and by creating special rules for marketing to small groups. The ASIM recommends converting Medicaid from a welfare program to a source of funding for all individuals who are unable to obtain employer-based health insurance, a mandated set of basic benefits under Medicaid, reform of physician payment to ensure adequate incentives for participation in Medicaid, and increased federal funding for Medicaid to reduce the financial burden on the states. The cost containment component calls for eliminating administrative hassles that impede access to care, reforming the medical liability system, requiring some patient cost sharing in all insurance plans, increasing research on the outcomes of different medical interventions, and developing practice guidelines to modify physician behavior and provide a basis for setting payment criteria. Further information can be obtained by writing to the American Society of Internal Medicine, 1101 Vermont Avenue N.W., Suite 500, Washington, DC 20005-3457.

have proposed legislation that would mandate employer-provided health care coverage for all workers and dependents (see box).

Legislative proposals to expand private health insurance would require employers to offer employees and dependents a health insurance plan that covers hospital care, physician care, and other needed services. The impact on adolescents could be significant, as almost 2 of 3 uninsured adolescents live in families where one or both parents work. However, its impact would depend on many factors, including the coverage offered to dependents and whether the mandate applied to all employers (including small businesses and the self-employed, part-time workers, and seasonal workers).

An analysis conducted for the Congressional Office of Technology Assessment estimated the effect of employer-mandated insurance using several assumptions:

- Self-employed persons would be exempt, but the mandate would otherwise apply to employers with firms of all sizes (71).

- Coverage would be offered to employees working more than 26 weeks per year (71).

- Dependents through 18 years of age who live with their parents would be covered as long as one parent was covered by the mandate (71).

If employees who worked 30 hours or more per week were included, approximately 2.5 million currently uninsured adolescents would be covered by the mandate, thus extending coverage to 55% of uninsured adolescents. An additional 200,000 adolescents would be covered if the mandate applied to all employees who worked 18 or more hours per week (71).

While legislation mandating employer health insurance coverage of employees and dependents has been introduced in Congress, no bills have been enacted so far. At the state level, Hawaii and Massachusetts have adopted laws mandating employer coverage of employees and their dependents, though only in Hawaii is the law fully operational. Other states are considering similar laws.

Combined Medicaid and Employer-Mandated Reforms

Employer mandates and Medicaid expansions have different effects on uninsured adolescents. The employer mandate would tend to benefit adolescents from lower- and middle-income families, while the Medicaid expansion would benefit the poor and near poor.

If Medicaid eligibility were set at 200% of the poverty level, and employers were mandated to provide coverage for employees working 18 or more hours per week, 99% of adolescents would have coverage. The remaining 1% would be primarily those adolescents living with parents who are self-employed (71). For this population, purchase of Medicaid or private insurance at subsidized rates could be considered.

Reducing High Out-of-Pocket Expenditures

If all adolescents were insured through Medicaid and employer-based private health insurance, some families would still pay substantial out-of-pocket expenses for adolescent medical care.

The single most important policy option for reducing high out-of-pocket costs is the provision of health insurance for all adolescents. It is critical that such coverage include comprehensive benefit plans and adequate catastrophic protection to meet the needs of all adolescents regardless of health status, family income, or source of insurance coverage. The elimination of catastrophic medical costs would require the use of income-adjusted premiums, deductibles, and coinsurance requirements so that a low-income family and a fam- ily with special health problems would not be disproportionately affected by cost-sharing requirements.

2. What other steps could ensure that adolescents receive needed health care services?

Much of the national debate on access to care focuses on (1) whether or not individuals have health insurance coverage, (2) the range of services included, and (3) the amount of money that a family or individual pays out of pocket for insurance premiums, copayment, or other costs of medical care. While these steps would substantially improve access to care for adolescents, other nonfinancial barriers to care still need to be addressed. This section reviews changes that would further enhance adolescents' access to quality care and provides examples of programs or projects that have been initiated to meet adolescent health needs. Addressed are the development of comprehensive and coordinated health care services for adolescents, the need for confidential care, changes in the training of medical and other health professionals, and the development of programs that promote adolescent health and responsible decision-making skills.

Comprehensive and coordinated care efforts sponsored by the Robert Wood Johnson Foundation

For more than 5 years, the Robert Wood Johnson Foundation funded 21 teaching hospitals and 54 community cosponsors to provide medical services and train health providers serving youth living in communities characterized by high rates of adolescent pregnancy, sexually transmitted disease, drug abuse, alcohol abuse, injury, homicide, suicide, and mental illness. The goals of the Program to Consolidate Services for High-Risk Young People were (a) to increase health services to high-risk youth; (b) to train health professionals caring for this population; (c) to consolidate categorical health services into a comprehensive care center; and (d) to secure long-term funding for adolescent health services (73).

The Robert Wood Johnson Foundation has also provided grants to enable states and localities to change the financing, organization, and delivery of mental health services. One change recommended by the Robert Wood Johnson Foundation is increasing available services by blending mental health, education, juvenile justice, and child welfare resources in which there are joint agency responsibilities. A second recommended change involves restructuring administrative and fiscal relationships between state and local government agencies. This would provide greater flexibility and incentives for expanding the range of services, with the development, for example, of single points of fiscal and program authority or county and state cost-sharing arrangements (66).

Comprehensive, Coordinated Care

Strong consensus exists that adolescents, especially those at high risk for health problems, would benefit greatly from comprehensive and coordinated health care. Comprehensive care refers to periodic preventive health services and screening, as well as treatment and referral for specific services such as mental health, substance abuse, family planning, and chronic illness and disability.

Some comprehensive adolescent health programs have sought to provide all services in a single site; other programs offer multisite services. Current models of comprehensive adolescent health services vary widely in their organization, funding sources, services provided, staff composition, and population served. The intent of these programs, however, is to provide direct care to adolescents who might otherwise not receive necessary services and to make it as easy as possible for them to receive services by the use of flexible hours, sliding fee scales, and improved staff rapport with adolescents.

The Maternal and Child Health Bureau (MCHB), which is part of the Department of Health and Human Services, has funded several projects in comprehensive community-based services for adolescents. The MCHB has also funded projects for adolescents in health promotion, teen pregnancy prevention, and adolescents with special health care needs, including those making the transition to adulthood. In addition, the MCHB funds research and training projects. A list of program abstracts appears in *Adolescent Health: Abstracts of Active Projects FY 1990*. A copy of the volume and other publications on adolescent health can be obtained by writing to the National Maternal and Child Health Clearinghouse (NMCHC), 38th and R Streets N.W., Washington, DC 20057.

Other local programs have been developed to serve adolescents considered to be at high risk because of poverty, violence, and other problems in their communities, or because they had begun to engage in health-threatening behaviors. One series of initiatives has been sponsored by the Office for Substance Abuse Prevention (OSAP). OSAP has funded prevention and intervention programs targeting high-risk youth in more than 130 communities in the United States. The funded programs establish linkages with public- and private-sector agencies and organizations to facilitate collaboration and comprehensive approaches to alcohol and other drug problems.

OSAP has recently published two volumes targeting high-risk youth and the environments in which they live. *Breaking New Ground for Youth at Risk: Program Summaries*

Local coordinating health councils

In 1990, the National Commission on the Role of the School and the Community in Improving Adolescent Health (funded by the Centers for Disease Control and sponsored by the AMA and the National Association of State Boards of Education) issued a report entitled *Code Blue: Uniting for Healthier Youth.* The Commission recommended the development of local councils that would coordinate health and social services for their areas. The local council would be composed of elected officials, agency heads, school and public health officials, private service providers, civic, business, and religious leaders, family members, and youth. They would have the power to investigate allegations of poor service and to conduct public hearings. The council would be recognized by the state as responsible for planning and implementing public and private interagency initiatives supporting the health and well-being of children, adolescents, and families. The coordinating council would develop long- and short-term goals, monitor the provision of services, develop systems to measure whether the goals are achieved, create an inventory of existing and needed services, encourage interagency collaboration and cooperation, develop protocols for case management, and stimulate and support neighborhood initiatives promoting adolescent health, including early support for families in trouble.

An example of a local coordinating council exists in Minneapolis. Since 1986, the Minneapolis Youth Coordinating Board (MYCB) has focused on the delivery of comprehensive services to children and adolescents. Since it began, the MYCB has directed several programs and collaborated on more than 30 others. Accomplishments include the expansion of health clinic services to all students attending Minneapolis public high schools, intervention in gang activities, and a diverse array of projects involving adolescents in community service, crime prevention, and a Twin Cities Youth Policy Forum. For further information, contact Colleen Walker, Director of Communications, Minnesota Youth Coordinating Board, 202 City Hall, Minneapolis, MN 55415.

reviews demonstration projects that were funded in 1987 to develop, test, and evaluate innovative prevention, intervention, and treatment approaches for high-risk youth. The book includes descriptions of programs designed especially for Asians/Pacific Islanders, blacks, Hispanics, Native Americans, white Americans, and multiethnic minorities. *Prevention Plus II: Tools for Creating and Sustaining Drug-Free Communities* is intended to help communities adopt a comprehensive systems approach to prevention. A copy of these volumes can be obtained by writing the National Clearinghouse for Alcohol and Drug Information, P.O. Box 2345, Rockville, MD 20852.

While high-risk adolescents clearly need primary and secondary health care services, it is important that all adolescents have access to comprehensive care. At a minimum, this will entail greater coordination between problem-specific or categorical programs. An even bolder initiative calls for fundamental change in the coordination of health care delivery through local coordinating councils.

Confidential Care

In 1989, the American College of Obstetricians and Gynecologists (ACOG) issued a policy statement on confidential health care for adolescents. The American Academy of Family Physicians, the American Academy of Pediatrics, the National Medical Association, and the Organization for Obstetric, Gynecologic, and Neonatal Nurses also approved the statement, which provides the following recommendations:

"Health professionals have an ethical obligation to provide the best possible care and counseling to respond to the needs of their adolescent patients. This obligation includes every reasonable effort to encourage the adolescent to involve parents, whose support can, in many circumstances, increase the potential for dealing with the adolescent's problems on a continuing basis. Parents are frequently in a patient relationship with the same providers as their children or have been exercising decision-making responsibility for their children with these providers. At the time providers establish an independent relationship with adolescents as

Highlights of AMA policy recommendations on confidential care

The information disclosed to a physician during the course of the relationship between physician and patient is confidential to the greatest possible degree. The patient should feel free to make a full disclosure of information to the physician in order that the physician may most effectively provide needed services. The patient should be able to make this disclosure with the knowledge that the physician will respect the confidential nature of the communication. The physician should not reveal confidential communications or information without the express consent of the patient, unless required to do so by law (18).

The AMA continues to oppose regulations that require parental notification when prescription contraceptives are provided to minors through federally funded programs, since they create a breach of confidentiality in the physician-patient relationship (21). The teenage girl whose sexual behavior exposes her to possible conception should have access to medical consultation and the most effective contraceptive advice and methods consistent with her physical and emotional needs. The physician should be free to prescribe or withhold contraceptive advice in accordance with his or her best medical judgment in the best interests of the patient (19). Obstacles to the distribution of birth control information, medication, and devices should be removed, and physicians should provide contraceptive services on a confidential basis where legally permissible (20).

patients, the providers should make this new relationship clear to parents and adolescents with regard to the following elements:

(a) The adolescent will have an opportunity for examination and counseling apart from parents, and the same confidentiality will be preserved between the adolescent patient and the provider as between the parent/adult and the provider.

(b) The adolescent must understand under what circumstances (e.g., life-threatening emergency) the provider will abrogate this confidentiality.

(c) Parents should be encouraged to work out means to facilitate communication regarding appointments, payment, or other matters consistent with the understanding reached about confidentiality and parental support in this transitional period when the adolescent is moving toward self-responsibility for health care.

(d) Providers, parents, and adolescents need to be aware of the nature and effect of laws and regulations in their jurisdictions that introduce further constraints on these relationships. Some of these laws and regulations are unduly restrictive and in need of revision as a matter of public policy. Ultimately, the health risks to the adolescents are so impelling that legal barriers and deference to parental involvement should not stand in the way of needed health care" (9).

The American College of Physicians (ACP) has also developed a position on patient-provider confidentiality. According to the ACP, "Caring for the adolescent patient typically occurs in the context of his or her family. It requires an understanding of the family dynamics of which the patient is a part. Family involvement, however, must be balanced with confidentiality needs and the right of the adolescent to exercise autonomy and self-determination in health care decisions and in his or her relationships with health care providers. Legislatures and courts vary in the amount of decision-making freedom (without parental consent or knowledge) they permit minors. [Physicians] should be aware of the relevant laws in their state" (10).

Professional Training and Clinical Practice

Change is needed in the training of physicians and other health professionals who work with adolescents. Information about and experience with adolescents should be increasingly incorporated into graduate and professional training as well as continuing education programs. Training should involve multiple disciplines. To provide the best possible care, health professionals need to improve their skills in the recognition, treatment, and referral of adolescents with complex psychosocial problems. Preventive interventions should be emphasized when appropriate (see box).

There are several projects designed to improve the training and clinical practice of health professionals working with adolescents. A sample of these projects includes the following:

The federal government has published clinical guidelines to address the uncertainty among clinicians about what preventive services should be offered to adolescents. In 1990, the U.S. Preventive Services Task Force issued a report, *Guide to Clinical Preventive Services* (U.S. Preventive Services Task Force, 1989), that contains guidelines to help health practitioners prevent 169 medical disorders and health problems. The guide was published after 4 years of study and was com-missioned by the Office of Disease Prevention and Health Promotion. The guide does not address all adolescent disorders and conditions, but its recommendations provide an important first step toward identifying problems that could be addressed during an office visit to a physician.

The AMA has been funded by the Centers for Disease Control, Division of Adolescent and School Health, to develop *Guidelines for Adolescent Preventive Services (GAPS)*. The guidelines will concern both organic and behavioral issues and will address the periodicity and content of preventive health services for adolescents. Further information can be obtained by writing the Department of Adolescent Health, American Medical Association, 515 N. State Street, Chicago, IL 60610.

The American Academy of Pediatrics (AAP) sponsors activities including continuing medical education courses, office-based research, conferences, and public education initiatives designed to improve the training and clinical practice of pediatricians who provide care for adolescents. The AAP has developed publications and manuals on substance abuse, sports medicine, school health, and other issues for practicing physicians. Further information can be obtained by writing the Division of Child and Adolescent Health, American Academy of Pediatrics, 141 Northwest Point Road, P.O. Box 927, Elk Grove Village, IL 60007.

Professional training in adolescent health and preventive medicine

A 1986 study group funded by the federal Maternal and Child Health Bureau and sponsored by the Society for Adolescent Medicine and the University of Minnesota focused on training health professionals in adolescent health care. The study group recommended that entry-level training for health professionals include (1) interdisciplinary training, (2) a curriculum including basic psychosocial maturation and normal adolescent growth as well as factors that predispose adolescents to health-threatening behavior, (3) developing the communication and problem-solving skills of health professionals working with adolescents and their families, (4) familiarity with community services and resources to make appropriate referrals, and (5) a self-assessment of the professional's own attitudes and values regarding adolescence (32).

A report by the U.S. Preventive Services Coordinating Committee noted that education and training programs in medicine need to include more information and learning experiences about prevention. Because many health-promoting or health-threatening behaviors begin during adolescence, it is important that physicians receive adequate training in preventive medicine as it pertains to adolescents. During the 1980s, only 61% of primary care residency programs provided seminars or lectures in preventive medicine, fewer than 2% of full-time faculty positions in undergraduate medical education were filled by preventive medicine or public health faculty, and fewer than 2% of U.S. medical school graduates had taken an elective in preventive medicine. The Coordinating Committee recommended that health promotion and disease prevention be taught throughout all phases of medical education (37).

The American College of Obstetricians and Gynecologists recently published a two-volume guide entitled *Adolescent Sexuality: Guides for Professional Involvement*. The guide includes material for lectures and presentations on adolescent sexuality and family life. Also included are articles, fact sheets, references, slides, sample handouts, and supplementary material. The guide can be purchased from the ACOG Distribution Center, P.O. Box 91180, Washington, DC 20090 (item No. AA106, parts 1 and 2).

Project Prevention, initiated by the American Academy of Child and Adolescent Psychiatry (AACAP), is a 2-year effort focusing on the prevention of mental illness in children and adolescents. The project has produced two major documents: a scientific report on prevention and an advocacy training report including 45 practical recommendations for child and adolescent psychiatrists. Further information about AACAP's Project Prevention can be obtained by writing the American Academy of Child and Adolescent Psychiatry, 3615 Wisconsin Avenue N.W., Washington, DC 20016.

The Handbook on Psychiatric Practice in the Juvenile Court is a product of an interdisciplinary work group established by the American Psychiatric Association. The volume should be a useful adjunct to training mental health professionals for work in the juvenile courts and should be of value to the legal profession as well. Further information can be obtained by writing to American Psychiatric Press, Inc.,

1400 K Street N.W., Washington, DC 20005.

To reduce preventable death, disease, and disability, the U.S. Public Health Service recently released *Healthy People 2000: National Health Promotion and Disease Prevention Objectives*. Of the almost 300 objectives, 45 target adolescents directly and another 51 affect adolescents as part of the broader population. A subset of these objectives pertain directly to health care professionals working with adolescents. The AMA, with funding from the Office of Disease Prevention and Health Promotion, has produced *Healthy Youth 2000: National Health Promotion and Disease Prevention Objectives for Adolescents*. The 50-page volume covers the objectives in 16 topic areas, contains additional objectives regarding the roles of health care professionals, schools, communities, and the government, and includes a set of Healthy People 2000 Resources. A copy of *Healthy Youth 2000* can be obtained by writing Betsy J. Davis, Department of Adolescent Health, American Medical Association, 515 N. State Street, Chicago, IL 60610.

The Society for Adolescent Medicine (SAM), a multidisciplinary organization, is devoted to the development of comprehensive acute, chronic, and preventive health care delivery to youth and to the scientific research regarding all aspects of adolescence. SAM publishes the *Journal of Adolescent Health* and holds an annual meeting to discuss scientific, training, and clinical practice issues related to the care of adolescents. Further information can be obtained by writing Edie Moore, 19401 East 40 Highway, Suite 120, Independence, MO 64055.

In 1990, the federal Maternal and Child Health Bureau (MCHB) funded the University of Cincinnati Adolescent Health Training Program to provide continuing education that meets the training needs of care providers. This will be accomplished by developing curricula to educate local providers about adolescent health issues. Plans for the project also include the development and implementation of a "train the trainer" curriculum to disseminate the adolescent health curricula. These trainers will plan, conduct, and evaluate a minimum of 24 workshops in the Midwest for providers of primary care to adolescents. For further information, contact Linda S. Wildey, Children's Hospital Medical Center, Adolescent Medicine, Elland and Bethesda Avenues, Cincinnati, OH 45229-2899.

MCHB also supports Resources for Enhancing Adolescent Community Health (REACH), a national resource for technical assistance to state maternal and child health agencies. The project's goal is to improve adolescent health status by increasing states' capacities to facilitate local action and to prevent and/or reduce adolescent health problems. To meet this goal, REACH will prepare a national database on community development in adolescent health that will be accessible through MCH-Net, a computer bulletin board. REACH will provide technical assistance and

consultation to states and communities and training to meet specific needs in selected states. For further information, contact Barbara S. Ritchen, Adolescent Health, Colorado Department of Health, 4210 East 11th Avenue, Denver, CO 80220-3716.

Health Education and Decision-Making Skills

Innovative programs that teach adolescents to make appropriate, health-promoting decisions are needed. It is especially important to find ways to help underserved, disenfranchised, and disabled adolescents. These programs should be adapted for multiple settings, including schools, office-based practices, and correctional institutions.

In 1990 the Carnegie Council on Adolescent Development published a report, *Life Skills Training: Preventive Interventions for Young Adolescents*. The report describes core elements of life skills training, including decision-making skills, problem solving, communication skills, impulse control, and social skills that help adolescents respond appropriately, particularly when confronted with use of drugs and alcohol, delinquency, early sexual involvement, and aggressive behaviors. The report highlights exemplary interventions based in schools, communities, and new conceptual models. A copy of the report can be obtained by writing to the Carnegie Council on Adolescent Development, 2400 N Street N.W., Washington, DC 20037-1153.

Between 1982 and 1988, the life and health insurance industry, along with the Robert Wood Johnson Foundation and the Henry J. Kaiser Family Foundation, supported INSURE, a study of prevention in primary care to determine whether preventive services could reduce the risk of disease and promote health. Adolescents between 12 and 17 years of age who participated in the prevention program showed no change in the rate of cigarette smoking, but the smoking rate was more than one-third higher among adolescents in the control group. Consumption of alcohol increased 5% among the study group but increased 15% among adolescents in the control group. Two thirds of physicians reported that as a result of the project they felt better prepared and more effective in educating their patients about reducing risk factors (74). The results of this project suggest that prevention in the primary care setting may deter some adolescents from becoming involved in health-threatening behavior but with less success among adolescents who are already participating in unhealthy behavior.

Summary and Implications

The delivery of health services to adolescents poses serious challenges to the U.S. health care system. Adolescents need services that tend to be inadequately insured and often unavailable, including pre-

ventive care, treatment for mental disorders and substance abuse services, reproductive care, and dental services. At the same time that their health-risk behaviors are increasing, many adolescents experience discontinuity of health providers, switching from a pediatrician to an internist or general practitioner. Many delay seeking care and avoid advice or guidance. Their providers often have limited training in adolescence or insufficient time to handle the special needs of adolescents.

There are several policy alternatives that would improve our current system of financing health care for uninsured and underinsured adolescents. To date, limited progress has been achieved in financial reform that will have a positive impact on adolescents and their health needs. Yet, indicators of health status, health services use, and health insurance status suggest that the new decade must be one in which we respond to the serious and growing needs of today's youth. Financial and nonfinancial barriers must be removed to ensure that adolescents have access to and use health services that appropriately address their health care needs.

Bibliography

1   Adams, P. F., & Hardy, A. M. (1989). *Current estimates from the National Health Interview Survey, 1988.* Vital and Health Statistics, Series 10, No. 173 (DHHS Publication No. 89-1501). Hyattsville, MD: National Center for Health Statistics.

2   Adger, H., Jr., McDonald, E. M., & DeAngelis, C. (1990). Substance abuse education in pediatrics. *Pediatrics, 86,* 555-560.

3   Alan Guttmacher Institute. (1981). *Teenage pregnancy: The problem that hasn't gone away.* New York: Alan Guttmacher Institute.

4   Alpert, J. J. (1990). Primary care: The future for pediatric education. *Pediatrics, 86,* 653-659.

5   American Academy of Family Physicians. (1991). *Age charts for periodic health examination.* Reprint No. 510. Kansas City, MO: American Academy of Family Physicians.

6   American Academy of Pediatrics Committee on Adolescence. (1989). Health care for children and adolescents in detention centers, jails, lock-ups, and other court-sponsored residential facilities. *Pediatrics, 84,* 1118-1120.

7   American Academy of Pediatrics Committee on Psychosocial Aspects of Child & Family Health. (1988). *Guidelines for health supervision II.* Elk Grove Village, IL: American Academy of Pediatrics.

8   American Academy of Pediatrics Council on Child and Adolescent Health. (1988). Age limits in pediatrics. *Pediatrics, 81,* 736.

9   American College of Obstetricians and Gynecologists. (1988). *ACOG statement of policy: Confidentiality in adolescent health care.* Washington, DC: American College of Obstetricians and Gynecologists.

10 American College of Physicians. (1989). Health care needs of the adolescent. *Annals of Internal Medicine, 110,* 930-935.

11 American Medical Association. (1990). *AMA model state bill to create a blue ribbon panel to study the physical and mental health care needs of detained and incarcerated youths.* Prepared by the AMA Department of State Legislation. Chicago: American Medical Association.

12 American Medical Association. (1988). *Survey of physician perceptions, attitudes, and practice behaviors concerning adolescent alcohol use.* Chicago: American Medical Association.

13 AMA Council on Long Range Planning and Development. (1989). *The environment of medicine.* Chicago: American Medical Association.

14 AMA Council on Scientific Affairs. (1989). Health care needs of homeless and runaway youths. *Journal of the American Medical Association, 262,* 1358-1361.

15 AMA Council on Scientific Affairs. (1989). Health status of youth in correctional facilities. *Journal of the American Medical Association, 263,* 987-991.

16 AMA Council on Scientific Affairs. (1983). Medical evaluations of healthy persons. *Journal of the American Medical Association, 249,* 1626-1633.

17 AMA Council on Scientific Affairs. (1989). Providing medical services through school-based health programs. *Journal of the American Medical Association, 261,* 1939-1942.

18 AMA Division of Communications. (1988). *Reference guide to policy and official statements.* Chicago: American Medical Association.

19 AMA House of Delegates. (1971, June). *Report I: Teenage pregnancy* (p. 56). Chicago: American Medical Association.

20 AMA House of Delegates. (1971, June). *Report 82: Family Planning* (p. 295). Chicago: American Medical Association.

21 AMA House of Delegates. (1983, December). *Resolution 65: Opposition to HHS regulations on contraceptive services to minors* (p. 291). Chicago: American Medical Association.

22 American School Health Association, Association for the Advancement of Health Education, & Society for Public Health Education, Inc. (1989). *The national adolescent student health survey: A report on the health of America's youth.* Oakland, CA: Third Party Publishing Company.

23 Anglin, T. (1991). Personal communication between Trina Anglin of Cleveland Metropolitan Hospital and Arthur B. Elster of the American Medical Association, January 1991.

24 Anno, B. J. (1984). The availability of health services for juvenile offenders: Preliminary results of a national survey. *Journal of Prison and Jail Health, 4,* 77-91.

25 Bachman, J. G., Johnston, L. D., & O'Malley, P. M. (1986). *Monitoring the future: Questionnaire responses from the nation's high school seniors, 1986.* Ann Arbor: University of Michigan.

26 Bacon, K. H. (1990, October 29). Children, elderly to receive increased Medicaid benefits. *Wall Street Journal,* p. A6.

27 Barrett, M. E., Simpson, D. D., & Lehman, W. E. (1988). Behavioral changes of adolescents in drug abuse prevention programs. *Journal of Clinical Psychology, 44,* 461-473.

28 Bastien, R. T., & Adelman, H. S. (1984). Noncompulsory versus legally mandated placement, perceived choice, and response to treatment among adolescents. *Journal of Consulting and Clinical Psychology, 22,* 171-179.

29 Bloom, B. (1990). Health insurance and medical care: Health of our nation's children, United States, 1988. In *Advance data from vital and health statistics,* No. 188 (DHHS Publication No. PHS 90-1250). Hyattsville, MD: National Center for Health Statistics.

30 Blum, R. W. (1987). Physicians' assessment of deficiencies and desire for training in adolescent care. *Journal of Medical Education, 62*, 401-407.

31 Blum, R. W., & Bearinger, L. H. (1990). Knowledge and attitudes of health professionals toward adolescent health care. *Journal of Adolescent Health Care, 11*, 289-294.

32 Blum, R., & Smith, M. (1988). Training of health professionals in adolescent health care: Study group report. *Journal of Adolescent Health Care, 9*, 46S-50S.

33 Burns, B. J. (1991). Mental health service use by adolescents in the 1970s and 1980s. *Journal of the American Academy of Child and Adolescent Psychiatry, 30*, 144-150.

34 Casamassimo, P. S., & Castaldi, C. R. (1982). Considerations in the management of the adolescent. *Pediatric Clinics of North America, 29*, 631-651.

35 Centers for Disease Control. (1991, February). *HIV/AIDS Surveillance Report*. Atlanta: Centers for Disease Control.

36 Chamie, M., Eisman, S., Forrest, J. D., Orr, M. T., & Torres, A. (1982). Factors affecting adolescents' use of family planning clinics. *Family Planning Perspectives, 14*, 126-182.

37 Chin, L., & Johnson, K. (1990). *The current status of preventive medicine in medical education: A review of the literature*. Draft background paper prepared for the U.S. Preventive Services Coordinating Committee. Washington, DC: Office of Disease Prevention and Health Promotion.

38 Darnton, N. (1989, July 31). Committed youth. *Newsweek*.

39 DiCarlo, S., & Gabel, J. (1988, November). Conventional health plans: A decade later. In *Research Bulletin*. Washington, DC: Health Insurance Association of America.

40 Dryfoos, J. (1990). *Adolescents at risk: Prevalence and prevention*. New York: Oxford University Press.

41 Dryfoos, J. (1988). *Putting the boys in the picture: A review of programs to promote sexual responsibility among young males*. Santa Cruz, CA: Network Publications.

42 DuRant, R. (1991). Overcoming barriers to adolescents' access to health care. In Hendee, W. R. (Ed.), *The health of adolescents*. San Francisco: Jossey-Bass.

43 Elkind, D. (1985). Cognitive development and adolescent disabilities. *Journal of Adolescent Health Care, 6*, 84-89.

44 English, A. (1985). Ensuring access to health care for teenagers: Legal and ethical issues concerning consent and confidentiality. *Youth Law News, 6*, 4-5, 22-24.

45 Felice, M. E. (1986). Reflections on caring for Indochinese children and youths. *Developmental and Behavioral Pediatrics, 7*, 124-128.

46 Fox, H. (1990, January 12). *1989 legislative amendments affecting access to care by children and pregnant women*. Memorandum to State Directors of Maternal and Child Health Services and Programs for Children With Special Health Needs and Other Interested Persons.

47 Fox, H., & Newacheck, P. (1990). Private health insurance of chronically ill children. *Pediatrics, 85*, 50-57.

48 Fox, H., Wicks, L., McManus, M., & Kelly, R. (1990, May). *Medicaid financing for mental health and substance abuse prevention and treatment services for children and adolescents*. Contract report prepared for the Alcohol, Drug Abuse and Mental Health Administration.

49 Fox, H., & Yoshpe, R. (1986, March). *Private health insurance coverage of chronically ill children*. Report prepared for the Future Directions of Services Project, National Maternal and Child Health Resource Center. Iowa City: University of Iowa.

50 Gans, J. E., Blyth, D. A., Elster, A. B., & Gaveras, L. L. (1990). *America's adolescents: How healthy are they?* Chicago: American Medical Association.

51 Gittler, J., Quigley-Rick, M., & Saks, M. J. (1990). *Adolescent health care decision making: The law and public policy*. Paper prepared with the support of the Carnegie Corporation of New York as a background paper for the United States Congress Office of Technology Assessment's Adolescent Health Project.

52 Grembowski, D., Andersen, R. M., & Chen, M. (1989). A public health model of the dental care process. *Medical Care Review, 46*, 439-496.

53 Gross, J. (1989, July 23). Homes for unwed mothers. *New York Times*, pp. 1, 25.

54 Gross, R. (1991, February). Personal communication between Richard L. Gross of the George Washington University School of Medicine and Janet E. Gans of the American Medical Association, February 1991.

55 Harrison, P. A., & Hoffman, N. G. (1989). *CATOR Report*. Unpublished manuscript.

56 Harvey, L. K., & Shubat, S. C. (1989). *Physician and public attitudes on health care issues, 1989 edition*. Chicago: American Medical Association.

57 Hein, K., Cohen, M. I., Litt, I. F., Schonberg, S. K., Meyer, M. R., Marks, A., & Sheehy, A. J. (1980). Juvenile detention: Another boundary issue for physicians. *Pediatrics, 66*, 239-245.

58 Henshaw, S. K., Forrest, J. D., & Van Vort, J. (1987). Abortion services in the United States, 1984 and 1985. *Family Planning Perspectives, 19*, 63-70.

59 Henshaw, S. K., Kenney, A. M., Somberg, D., & Van Vort, J. (1989). *Teenage pregnancy in the United States: The scope of the problem and state responses*. New York: Alan Guttmacher Institute.

60 Hofmann, A. D. (1983). Legal issues in adolescent medicine. In Hofmann, A. D. (Ed.), *Adolescent medicine*. Menlo Park, CA: Addison-Wesley.

61 Hughes, D., Johnson, K., Rosenbaum, S., Butler, E., & Simons, J. (1988). *The health of America's children: Maternal and child health data book*. Washington, DC: Children's Defense Fund.

62 Hyche-Williams, H. J., & Waszak, C. (1991). *School-based clinics: Update 1990*. Washington, DC: Center for Population Options.

63 Irwin, C. E., Jr. (1991). Personal communication between Charles E. Irwin, Jr., of the University of California-San Francisco Medical Center and Arthur B. Elster of the American Medical Association, January 1991.

64 Irwin, C. E., Jr. (1986). Why adolescent medicine? *Journal of Adolescent Health Care, 7*, 2S-12S.

65 Jack, S., & Bloom, B. (1988). *Use of dental services and dental health, United States: 1986*. Vital and Health Statistics, Series 10, No. 165 (DHHS Publication No. PHS 88-1593). Hyattsville, MD: National Center for Health Statistics.

66 Jacobs, J. H. (1990). Child mental health: Service system and policy issues. *Social Policy Report, 4*, 1-18.

67 Jenks, B., Polizos, V., & Gotlieb, E. (1988). Health care in juvenile justice facilities in Georgia. *Journal of the Medical Association of Georgia, 77*, 775-778.

68 Kamerow, D. B., Pincus, H. A., & McDonald, D. I. (1986). Alcohol abuse, other drug abuse, and mental disorders in medical practice. *Journal of the American Medical Association, 255*, 2054-2057.

69 Kirby, D., Waszak, C. S., & Ziegler, J. (1989). *An assessment of six school-based clinics: Services, impact and potential*. Washington, DC: Center for Population Options.

70 Kozak, L. J., Norton, C., McManus, M., & McCarthy, E. (1987). Hospital use patterns for children in the United States, 1983 and 1984. *Pediatrics, 80*, 481-490.

71 Kronick, R. (1989). *Adolescent health insurance status: Analysis of trends in coverage and preliminary estimates of the effects of an employer mandate and Medicaid expansion on the uninsured*. Report prepared for the U.S. Congress Office of Technology Assessment. Washington, DC: U.S. Government Printing Office.

72 Lear, J. G. (1989). The school-based adolescent health care program: Reaching teenagers where teenagers are. In *Proceedings from the 1989 Adolescent Health Coordinators Conference*. Washington, DC: National Center for Education in Maternal and Child Health.

73 Lear, J. G., Foster, H. W., & Baratz, J. A. (1989). The high-risk young people's program: A summing up. *Journal of Adolescent Health Care, 10*, 224-230.

74 Logsdon, D. (1988). Unpublished report from the INSURE Project.

75 Lovett, J., & Wald, M. S. (1985). Physician attitudes toward confidential care for adolescents. *Journal of Pediatrics, 106*, 517-521.

76 Lovick, S., & Stern, R. F. (1988). *School-based clinics: Update 1988*. Washington, DC: Center for Population Options.

77 Malus, M., LaChance, P. A., Lamy, L., Macaulay, A., & Vanasse, M. (1987). Priorities in adolescent health care: The teenager's viewpoint. *Journal of Family Practice, 25*, 159-162.

78 Manson, S., & Bergeisen, L. (1990). *Indian adolescent mental health* (special report OTA-H-446). Report prepared by the U.S. Congress Office of Technology Assessment. Washington, DC: U.S. Government Printing Office.

79 Marks, A. M., & Fisher, M. F. (1987). Health assessment and screening during adolescence. *Pediatrics, 80 (Suppl.)*, 135-158.

80 Marks, A., Malizio, J., Hoch, J., Brody, R., & Fisher, M. (1983). Assessment of health needs and willingness to utilize health care resources of adolescents in a suburban population. *Journal of Pediatrics, 102*, 456-460.

81 McManus, M., Flint, S., & Kelly, R. (1991). The adequacy of physician reimbursement for pediatric care under Medicaid. *Pediatrics, 87*, in press.

82 McManus, M., McCarthy, E., Kozak, L. J., & Newacheck, P. (1991). Hospital use by adolescents and young adults. *Journal of Adolescent Health Care, 12*, 107-115.

83 McManus, M. A., Newacheck, P. W., & Weader, R. A. (1990). Metropolitan and nonmetropolitan adolescents: Differences in demographic and health characteristics. *Journal of Rural Health, 6*, 39-51.

84 Mitchell, J. (1988, November). *Mental health problems of incarcerated youth*. Paper presented at the AMA Working Group on the Health Status of Detained and Incarcerated Youth, Chicago, IL.

85 Moore, K. A. (1988). *Facts at a glance*. Washington, DC: Child Trends.

86 Moore, K., & Burt, M. (1982). *Private crisis, public cost: Policy perspectives on teenage childbearing*. Washington, DC: Urban Institute.

87 Mosher, W. D. (1990, April). Use of family planning services in the United States: 1982 and 1988. In *Advance data from vital and health statistics*, No. 184 (DHHS Publication No. PHS 90-1250). Hyattsville, MD: National Center for Health Statistics.

88 National Advisory Mental Health Council. (1990). *National plan for research on child and adolescent mental disorders: A report requested by the U.S. Congress* (DHHS Publication No. ADM 90-1683). Washington, DC: U.S. Department of Health and Human Services.

89 National Association of Children's Hospitals and Related Institutions. (1990). *Kids' clout: Americans' attitudes on children's issues*. Alexandria, VA: National Association of Children's Hospitals and Related Institutions.

90 National Center for Health Statistics. (1990). *Advance report of final natality statistics, 1988*. Monthly Vital Statistics Report (Suppl.) (DHHS Publication No. 90-1120). Hyattsville, MD: National Center for Health Statistics.

91 National Center for Youth With Disabilities. (1989, spring/summer). *Connections*. Minneapolis: National Center for Youth With Disabilities.

92 National Conference of Commissioners on Uniform State Laws, Uniform Health-Care Information Act. (1988). *Uniform Laws Annotated, Part I* (9, pp. 475-520). St. Paul, MN: West Publishing Company.

93 National Conference of State Legislatures. (1989). *Coordinating child juvenile justice, mental health, and welfare systems.* Paper presented at the Conference on Treatment of Adolescents With Alcohol, Drug, and Mental Health Problems, Alexandria, VA.

94 National Institute on Drug Abuse. (1990). *Annual data 1989: Data from the Drug Abuse Warning Network (DAWN)*, Series I, No. 9 (DHHS Publication No. ADM 90-1717). Rockville, MD: National Institute on Drug Abuse.

95 National Institute on Drug Abuse. (1989). *National Drug and Alcoholism Treatment Unit Survey, 1987 final report* (DHHS Publication No. ADM 89-1626). Rockville, MD: U.S. Alcohol, Drug Abuse, and Mental Health Administration.

96 National Institute on Drug Abuse. (1989). *National household survey on drug abuse: Population estimates 1988* (DHHS Publication No. ADM 89-1636). Washington, DC: U.S. Government Printing Office.

97 National Mental Health Association. (1989). *Facts: Children with mental disorders.* Alexandria, VA: National Mental Health Association.

98 Neinstein, L. S., Shapiro, J., & Rabinovitz, S. (1986). Effect of an adolescent medicine rotation on medical students and pediatric residents. *Journal of Adolescent Health Care, 7,* 345-349.

99 Nelson, C. (1991). Office visits by adolescents. In *Advance data from vital and health statistics,* No. 196 (DHHS Publication No. PHS 87-1250). Hyattsville, MD: National Center for Health Statistics.

100 Newacheck, P. W. (1989). Adolescents with special health needs: Prevalence, severity, and access to health services. *Pediatrics, 84,* 872-881.

101 Newacheck, P. W., & McManus, M. A. (1990). Health care expenditure patterns for adolescents. *Journal of Adolescent Health Care, 11,* 133-140. Note: Dollar amounts in this article have been adjusted to 1990 dollars for this volume.

102 Newacheck, P. W., & McManus, M. A. (1989). Health insurance status of adolescents in the United States. *Pediatrics, 84,* 699-708.

103 Newacheck, P. W., & McManus, M. A. (1991). Original tabulations from the 1986 National Health Interview Survey.

104 Nidorf, J. F., & Morgan, M. C. (1987). Cross cultural issues in adolescent medicine. *Primary Care, 14,* 69-82.

105 Noble, J. (1989). *Reimbursement for adolescent alcohol, drug abuse, and mental health treatment.* Paper presented at the Conference on Treatment of Adolescents With Alcohol, Drug Abuse, and Mental Health Problems, Alexandria, VA.

106 Novack, D. H., Detering, B. J., Arnold, R., Forrow, L., Ladinsky, M., & Pezzullo, J. C. (1989). Physicians' attitudes toward using deception to resolve difficult ethical problems. *Journal of the American Medical Association, 261,* 2980-2985.

107 Office of Population Affairs. (1990). *The adolescent family life demonstration projects: Program and evaluation summaries 1989-1990 update.* Washington, DC: U.S. Department of Health and Human Services.

108 Orr, D. P., Weiser, S. P., Dian, D. A., & Maurana, C. A. (1987). Adolescent health care: Perception and needs of the practicing physician. *Journal of Adolescent Health Care, 8,* 239-245.

109 Perrin, J., Valvona, J., & Sloan, F. (1986). Changing patterns of hospitalization for children requiring surgery. *Pediatrics, 77,* 587-592.

110 Pfeiffer, S. I., & Strzelecki, S. C. (1990). Inpatient psychiatric treatment of children and adolescents: A review of outcome studies. *Journal of the American Academy of Child and Adolescent Psychiatry, 29,* 847-853.

111 Reis, J., Reid, E., Herr, T., & Herz, E. (1987, Winter). Family planning for inner-city adolescent males: Pilot study. *Adolescence, 23,* 953-960.

112 Resnick, M., Blum, R. W., & Hedlin, D. (1980). The appropriateness of health services for adolescents: Youths' opinions and attitudes. *Journal of Adolescent Health Care, 1,* 137-141.

113 Rosenbaum, S., & Johnson, K. (1986). Providing health care for low-income children: Reconciling child health goals with child health financing realities. *Milbank Quarterly, 64,* 442-478.

114 Saxe, L. M., Cross, T., & Silverman, N. (1986). *Children's mental health: Problems and services.* Report prepared for the U.S. Congress Office of Technology Assessment. Durham, NC: Duke University Press.

115 Schiffman, J. R. (1989, February 3). Children's wards: Teen-agers end up in psychiatric hospitals in alarming numbers. *Wall Street Journal,* p. 1.

116 Shafer, M. A., & Moscicki, A. B. (1991). Sexually transmitted diseases in adolescents. In Hendee, W. R. (Ed.), *The health of adolescents.* San Francisco: Jossey-Bass.

117 Siegel, D. M. (1987). Adolescents and chronic illness. *Journal of the American Medical Association, 275,* 3396-3399.

118 Silber, T. J. (1986). Approaching the adolescent patient: Pitfalls and solutions. *Journal of Adolescent Health Care, 7,* 31S-40S.

119 Smith, M. J., & Grow, L. J. (1971). *Services to unmarried mothers in 1969.* New York: Child Welfare League of America.

120 Stone, R., & Waszak, C. (1989). *Teenage pregnancy and too-early childbearing: Public costs, personal consequences*. Washington, DC: Center for Population Options.

121 Stroup, A. L., Witkin, J. J., Atay, J. E., Fell, A. S., & Mandersheid, R. W. (1988). *Residential treatment centers for emotionally disturbed children, United States, 1983* (DHHS Publication No. ADM 88-1566). Rockville, MD: National Institute of Mental Health.

122 Swartz, D., & Darabi, L. (1984). *Why did you come to the clinic tonight? Motivations for adolescents' first visits to birth control clinics.* Paper presented at American Public Health Association, November.

123 Torres, A., & Forrest, J. D. (1988). Why do women have abortions? *Family Planning Perspectives, 20*, 169-176.

124 U.S. Congress Office of Technology Assessment (in press). *Adolescent health, volume 2: Background and effectiveness of selected prevention and treatment services* (Publication No. OTA-466). Washington, DC: U.S. Government Printing Office.

125 U.S. Congress Office of Technology Assessment. (1987, December). *Neonatal intensive care for low birthweight infants: Costs and effectiveness.* Health Technology Case Study No. 38 (Publication No. OTA-HCS-38). Washington, DC: U.S. Government Printing Office.

126 U.S. Department of Health, Education, and Welfare. (1979). *Healthy people: The surgeon general's report on health promotion and disease prevention background papers 1979* (DHEW Publication No. 79-55071A). Washington, DC: U.S. Government Printing Office.

127 U.S. Department of Health and Human Services. (1982). *Dental treatment needs of United States children 1979-1980* (NIH Publication No. 83-2246). Washington, DC: Government Printing Office.

128 U.S. Department of Health and Human Services. (1989). *Oral health of United States children: National and regional findings from the National Survey of Dental Caries in U.S. School Children, 1986-1987* (NIH Publication No. 98-2247). Bethesda, MD: National Institute for Dental Research.

129 U.S. Department of Justice. (1989). *Children in custody, 1975-85: Census of public and private juvenile detention, correctional, and shelter facilities* (Publication No. NCJ-114065). Washington, DC: Bureau of Justice Statistics.

130 U.S. General Accounting Office. (1989). *Health care: Home care experiences of families with chronically ill children* (Publication No. GAO/HRD-89-73). Gaithersburg, MD: U.S. General Accounting Office.

131 U.S. House of Representatives Select Committee on Children, Youth, and Families. (1985, August 14). *Opportunities for success: Cost effective programs for children.* Washington, DC: U.S. Government Printing Office.

132 U.S. Preventive Services Task Force. (1989). *Guide to clinical preventive services: An assessment of the effectiveness of 169 interventions.* Report of the U.S. Preventive Services Task Force. Baltimore, MD: Williams & Wilkins.

133 Vecchiolla, F. J., & Maza, P. L. (1989). *Pregnant and parenting adolescents: A study of services.* Washington, DC: Child Welfare League of America.

134 Waldo, D. R., Sonnefeld, S. T., McKusick, D. R., & Arnett, R. H. (1989). Health care financing trends: health care expenditures by age group, 1977 and 1987. *Health Care Financing Review, 10*, 111-120.

135 White-Means, S. T., & Thornton, M. C. (1989). Nonemergency visits to hospital emergency rooms: A comparison of blacks and whites. *Milbank Quarterly, 67*, 35-57.

136 Yudkowsky, B. K. (1990). Personal communication between Beth Yudkowsky of the American Academy of Pediatrics and Margaret McManus of McManus Health Policy, Inc., March 1990.

137 Yudkowsky, B. K., Cartland, J. D. C., & Flint, S. S. (1990). Pediatrician participation in Medicaid: 1978-1989. *Pediatrics, 85*, 567-577.

138 Yunker, R., Levine, M., & Sajid, A. (1988). Freestanding emergency centers and the health care of adolescents. *Journal of Adolescent Health Care, 9*, 321-324.

Index

Abortion 20

Abuse and neglect ix, 4, 24, 47, 51, 63

Access to care (see also Barriers to care, Health policy, Insurance, Private insurance, Public insurance) x
    American Academy of Family Physicians (AAFP) 60, 61
    American Academy of Pediatrics (AAP) 60
    American College of Physicians (ACP) 61
    American Medical Association (AMA) 60
    American Society of Internal Medicine (ASIM) 61
    availability of physicians 46
    chronic illness 21
    community size differences in 46
    comprehensive and coordinated care 2, 63, 65
    confidential care 66
    copayment 63
    data on 43
    decision-making skills 63
    Early and Periodic Screening, Diagnosis, and Treatment (EPSDT) Program 36
    emergency rooms 21
    health care financing xii, 61
    health policy xii, 36, 46, 61
    health promotion 47
    health services x, 46, 58, 70
    high-risk adolescents 65
    homeless adolescents 21
    insurance status x, xi, 21, 30, 43, 46, 63
    legal status of adolescents 66
    local coordinating councils 65
    Maternal and Child Health block grants 46
    maternity-related services 21, 46
    Medicaid xii, 30, 60, 61
    nonfinancial barriers to care 66
    out-of-pocket expenses 63
    poverty x, 30
    preventive care 36
    provider reimbursement xi
    routine health care 46
    Title V 46

Acute conditions x, 5, 23, 36, 40

Adoption 20

AIDS (see also HIV [human immuno-deficiency virus] infection, Sexually transmitted diseases [STDs]) 19, 25

Alaskan Native adolescents 16

Alcohol use
    among adolescents of all ages ix, 17, 19

female adolescents 18
health-threatening behaviors ix, 70
incarcerated adolescents 24
legal status of adolescents 53
male adolescents 18
mental health and disorders 14
patient-provider confidentiality 53
physician-patient communication 19, 55
physician visits 55

Alcohol abuse treatment services 17, 18
    comprehensive and coordinated care 47, 63
    cost of 42
    Drug Abuse Warning Network (DAWN) 22
    emergency room services 22
    health education 19, 69
    health services 47
    insurance coverage 19
    National Drug and Alcoholism Treatment Unit Survey 17
    out-of-pocket expenses 40
    outpatient services 18
    physician training 48, 49
    prevalence of 17
    psychiatric treatment 15
    referral services 19

American Academy of Child and Adolescent Psychiatry (AACAP) 68

American Academy of Family Physicians (AAFP) 5, 60, 61

American Academy of Pediatrics (AAP) 5, 51, 60, 67

American College of Obstetricians and Gynecologists (ACOG) 65, 68

American College of Physicians (ACP) 61, 66

American Medical Association (AMA)
    access to care 60
    adolescent medicine specialists 47
    confidential health services 53
    contraceptive use 65
    employer-mandated coverage 60
    Guidelines for Adolescent Preventive Services (GAPS) 67
    Health Access America 60
    health policy recommendations 5, 24-26, 60, 65
    health promotion and disease prevention 60
    homeless adolescents 26
    incarcerated adolescents 25
    legal status of adolescents 65
    Medicaid 60
    medical education 60
    parental notification 65
    patient-provider confidentiality 53, 65

physician attitudes toward alcohol use 19
physician training 67
school-based health centers 24
uninsured adolescents 60

American Psychiatric Association (APA) 68

American Society of Internal Medicine (ASIM) 61

Asian American adolescents 3

Barriers to care (see also Access to care, Health policy, Insurance)
    adolescent attitudes and behaviors 2
    adolescents' view of health care 56
    age differences in 2
    assessment of 1
    availability of physicians 46
    central-city adolescents 46
    chronic illness xi, 21, 50
    confidentiality xi, xiii, 46, 51, 54, 57, 66
    conflict with parents 54
    consequences of 54
    contraceptive use-related 54
    denial xii, 56
    depression 51
    disabled adolescents xi, xiii, 50
    drug abuse 51
    embarrassment xii, 56
    emergency rooms 21
    family planning clinics 20
    fear xii, 54
    financial xiii, 2, 56, 58, 70
    health education xiii, 56, 57
    health professionals 49
    health services 44, 46, 53, 70
    high-risk adolescents xi
    homeless adolescents xiii, 21, 25
    incarcerated adolescents xiii, 21, 24
    insurance xi, xiii, 21, 30, 46, 54
    lack of coordinated care xi, xiii, 46
    lack of knowledge xii, 54, 56
    legal status of adolescents 51
    male adolescents 54
    Maternal and Child Health block grants 46
    Medicaid 30
    minority adolescents xiii
    nonfinancial xi, xiii, 1, 2, 45, 53, 54, 55, 56, 57, 66, 70
    office setting 51
    parental consent/notification 56, 66
    patient compliance 57
    patient-provider communication xiii, 53, 55
    physician training xiii, 46, 49, 53, 57
    poverty 30
    pregnancy 21, 56
    psychosocial development issues 54

public clinics 21
reimbursement rates 30
routine health care 46
rural adolescents xiii, 46
scheduling of visits 51
sex education 56
sexual behavior 51
sexually transmitted diseases (STDs) 51, 56
substance abuse 56
time restraints 49
transportation 56

Black adolescents
    birth rates among ix
    dental visits 11
    family planning clinics 19
    homicide ix
    hospitalization 9
    insurance status 29, 31, 33
    mental health services 16
    older adolescents ix
    physician visits 6
    public clinic use 22
    reproductive health 19

Cancer 1

Carnegie Council on Adolescent Development 69

Case management xi, 16, 36, 64

Center for Population Options 42

Central-city adolescents 29, 33, 46

Child Welfare League of America (CWLA) 20

Childbirth (see Maternity-related services, Reproductive health)

Chronic illness (see also Disabled adolescents, Health policy, Insurance) 4, 5
    barriers to care xi, 21
    case management 50
    comprehensive and coordinated care xi, 50, 63
    data on 50
    definition of 5
    health needs of adolescents with 50
    high health care expenses 41
    hospitalization 26
    Koop, C. Everett 50
    life expectancy ix
    Medicaid 41
    out-of-pocket expenses 42
    physician training and knowledge about 50
    prevalence of 9, 26
    race differences in 26
    transition to adult health care system 50

Civilian Health and Medical Program of the Uniformed Services (CHAMPUS) 30

Cocaine ix

Code Blue: Uniting for Healthier Youth 64

Compliance xii

Comprehensive health services 36
    access to care 36, 65
    chronic illness 63
    definition of 63
    disabled adolescents 63
    family planning 63
    funding for 63
    health policy 36
    high-risk adolescents 63, 65
    homeless adolescents 25, 26
    Maternal and Child Health Bureau (MCHB) 64
    Robert Wood Johnson Foundation 63
    sliding fee scales 64
    substance abuse 63

Condoms 20

Confidentiality (see Patient-provider confidentiality)

Contraceptive use (see also Abortion, Adoption, Maternity-related services, Reproductive health)
    American Medical Association 65
    female adolescents 20
    health policy 65
    legal status of adolescents 65
    male adolescents 20
    patient-provider confidentiality 65
    physician visits 7, 52, 55
    school-based health centers 22

Coordinated care 2
    abuse and neglect 47
    access to care 46, 65
    alcohol abuse treatment services 47
    barriers to care xiii, 46, 47
    case management 64
    description of 63
    disabled adolescents 50
    fragmentation of 47
    health policy 36, 47, 63-65
    health services 16, 46, 47
    high-risk adolescents xi, 63, 65
    local coordinating councils 64
    Maternal and Child Health Bureau 64
    mental health services xi
    multiple health problems 47
    organization of 47
    pregnancy 47
    prevention and intervention 47, 64
    Robert Wood Johnson Foundation 63
    social services xi
    substance abuse treatment services xi, 47

Copayment 32, 34

Cost-sharing requirements xi, 1, 41, 61, 63

Death ix, 4, 25

Dental health (see also Orthodontists) 2,

4, 11, 12, 25, 36

Depression
    Alaskan Native and Native American adolescents 16
    incarcerated adolescents 24
    mental health services 16
    patient-provider communication 55
    physician training 48
    physician visits 51, 52, 55
    prevalence of 54
    sex differences in 54

Dermatologists 5, 8

Disabled adolescents (see also Chronic illness, Health policy, Insurance) ix
    barriers to care xiii, 50
    case management 50
    comprehensive and coordinated care xi, 50, 63
    health care financing 58
    health education 69
    health expenses 26, 41, 42, 50
    health needs of 50
    health services for xiii, 26
    high-risk pools 43
    hospitalization 26, 41
    insurance coverage x, 41, 43, 50
    life expectancy of xi
    Medicaid 41, 43
    medically uninsurable 43
    mental health ix
    outpatient care 41
    physician visits 26
    poverty 26
    preexisting conditions 43
    prevalence of 26
    race differences in 26
    state programs 41

Drug abuse 1, 51, 56

Drug Abuse Warning Network (DAWN) (see also Emergency rooms) 22

Ear, nose, and throat specialists 8

Early and Periodic Screening, Diagnosis, and Treatment (EPSDT) Program 36, 37

Emergency rooms 2, 4, 21, 22

Employer-mandated health insurance 59-62

Family planning (see also Contraceptive use, Maternity-related services, Reproductive health)
    barriers to care 20, 54
    comprehensive care 63
    condom distribution 20
    contraceptives 5, 20, 22
    coordinated care 63
    health expenses 37, 38
    health services 26
    inner-city 20
    older adolescents 19
    parental awareness of use 20

prevalence of use 20
race differences in 19
school-based health clinics 22
services for males 20
young adolescents 19

Family practitioners
age differences in visits to 8
physician training 47, 49
prevalence of visits to 8
trends in visits to 8

Female adolescents
abortion 19, 20
adoption 20
alcohol 18
contraceptive use 20, 54
depression 54
health expenses 37, 41
health services for 9, 11, 13, 14, 54
patient-provider communication 54
pregnancy and childbirth 19, 20
reproductive health 19, 37
sexual behavior 19, 54
sexually transmitted diseases 19
substance abuse treatment services 18

Financing (see Health care financing,
Health policy, Insurance, Medicaid)

Gingivitis 11

Guidelines for Adolescent Preventive
Services (GAPS) 67

Gynecologists (see also American College
of Obstetricians and Gynecologists
[ACOG]) 8, 9, 49

Health Access America 60

Health care financing (see also Health
policy, Insurance) xii, 58, 59, 61-63

Health education xiii, 5, 23, 57, 69

Health expenses (see also Barriers to
care, Health care financing, Health
policy, Insurance, Medicaid) 2, 3, 27, 37,
39, 41
age differences in 37
alcohol abuse-related 40
chronic illness 41
confidential services 38
cost-sharing requirements 41
data on 38
female adolescents 37
health services 42
hospitalization 37-39
income differences in 37, 39
insurance 38, 40, 42
limitations of data on 37, 38
long-term care 41
male adolescents 37
medical supplies and technology 38,
39
mental health services 37-41
National Medical Care Expenditure
Survey (NMCES) 38

National Medical Care Utilization and
Expenditure Survey (NMCUES) 38
National Medical Expenditure Survey
(NMES) 38
nonphysician services 39
out-of-pocket expenses 38, 40, 41
outpatient services 38, 39
physician services 39
poverty 37, 39, 41
prescription medicine 38, 39
preventive services 37, 38
race and ethnic differences in 37
reproductive health services 37, 38,
40, 42
risk for high expenses 41
sex differences in 37, 41
substance abuse treatment services 37,
40
underreporting of 38
uninsured adolescents 40

Health maintenance organizations
(HMOs) 32, 42

Health policy (see also Health care fi-
nancing, Insurance) 2
access to care 36, 46, 61
American Academy of Family
Physicians 61, 65
American Academy of Pediatrics 65
American College of Obstetricians and
Gynecologists 65
American College of Physicians 61
American Medical Association 5, 24,
65
American Society of Internal Medicine
61
barriers to care 45, 46
Code Blue: Uniting for Healthier Youth
64
contraceptive use 53, 65
coordinated care 47
Early and Periodic Screening,
Diagnosis, and Treatment (EPSDT)
Program 36
employer-mandated health insurance
61, 62
health care financing 58, 70
health services 53, 70
homeless adolescents 26
legal status of adolescents 53, 65, 66
local coordinating councils 64
long-term care 61
Maternal and Child Health block
grants 46
Medicaid xii, 35, 61
National Medical Association 65
Office of Substance Abuse Prevention
(OSAP) 65
Omnibus Budget Reconciliation Act of
1989 36
Organization for Obstetric,
Gynecologic, and Neonatal Nurses 65
parental consent/notification 52, 65, 66

patient-provider confidentiality 65, 66
preventive care 5
private insurance 61
public assistance 35, 61
public insurance 35
recommendations 5, 35, 62
state level 62
Title V 46
Title XX 21
underinsured adolescents 59
uninsured adolescents xiii, 34, 59
"working poor" 35

Health professionals xi, 1, 65
attitudes of 50
barriers to care xi, 49
clinical practice 50, 66
health policy 65
minority adolescents 50
non-Western medical practices 50
patient-provider communication 50
sensitivity of xii, 50
time restraints 49
training xi, 66

Health promotion
access to care 47
comprehensive care 64
coordinated care 64
health-threatening behaviors 67
Maternal and Child Health Bureau 64
maternity-related 64
physician training 67
prevention and intervention 5, 67

Health services (see also specific
services) ix, x, 1, 2, 3, 4, 27, 46
abortion 20
access to care x, 21, 46, 58, 60
adolescent attitudes toward xii, 52, 57
adolescent knowledge of 57
alcohol abuse treatment services 18,
47, 53
alternative health care sites 4, 21, 26
availability of 46
barriers to care 21, 44, 46, 54, 57
characteristics of 1, 57
Civilian Health and Medical Program
of the Uniformed Services (CHAMPUS)
30
comprehensive and coordinated care 1,
45-47, 64
contraceptive use 57
dental health 70
disabled adolescents 26
emergency rooms 21, 22
funding 46
geographic differences in 46
health expenses 38, 39
Health Maintenance Organizations
(HMOs) 42
health policy 53, 60
health promotion 46
homeless adolescents 4, 21, 25, 26
hospitalization 21, 37, 38

incarcerated adolescents 4, 21, 24, 25
income differences in use 46
insurance status x, 21, 26, 30, 46, 70
legal status of adolescents 51
Maternal and Child Health block
grants 46
maternity-related services 21, 42, 46,
47
Medicaid 30
mental health services 16, 37, 53, 70
minority adolescents 21, 26
organization of 46
parental involvement 52
patient compliance 57
patient-provider confidentiality 46, 52,
57
Preferred provider organizations
(PPOs) 42
prevention and intervention 26, 37, 47,
70
primary care physicians 46
public clinics 21
race and ethnic differences in 26
reproductive health care 19, 26, 42, 70
routine health care 43, 46
school-based health centers 21, 22
sexually transmitted diseases (STDs)
57
social services 21
substance abuse treatment services 18,
47, 53, 70
Title V 46

Health-threatening behavior (see also
High-risk adolescents) 1, 10
comprehensive care 64
coordinated care 64
homeless adolescents 26
Office for Substance Abuse
Prevention (OSAP) 64
prevention and intervention 4, 5, 67,
70
programs for 64
Robert Wood Johnson Foundation 70
trends in 4

Healthy People 2000 68

Healthy Youth 2000 68

Henry J. Kaiser Foundation 70

High-risk adolescents (see also Health-
threatening behavior) 1
access to care 63, 65
barriers to care xi, 54
comprehensive and coordinated care
xi, 63, 65
health services 70
poverty and violence 64
primary care 65
programs for 64
Robert Wood Johnson Foundation 63

Hispanic adolescents
dental visits 11
health services 43

hospitalization 9
insurance status 29, 31, 33, 43
limitations of data on 3
physician visits 6
poverty 43
preventive care 43
primary care 43
public clinic use 22

HIV (human immunodeficiency virus)
infection (see also AIDS, Sexually
transmitted diseases [STDs]) 19

HMO (see Health maintenance
organizations [HMOs])

Home health services xi

Homeless adolescents x, xiii, 4, 21, 25,
26

Homicide ix, 4

Hospitalization 2, 4, 5, 9
age differences in x, 9, 10
alcohol- and drug-related 11
disabled adolescents 26, 41
genitourinary diseases 10
geographic differences in 10
health expenses 37-39
income differences in 9
injury and poisoning 10
insurance status xi, 9, 10, 43
maternity-related services 10, 11
out-of-pocket expenses 40
prevalence of 9
psychiatric 10, 15
race and ethnic differences in 9
rates of x, 9, 10, 43
reasons for 5, 10
rural adolescents 9
sex differences in 9, 10, 11
sexually transmitted diseases 10
suicide-related 11
trends in 37
uninsured adolescents x

Incarcerated adolescents x, xi, xiii, 4, 21,
24, 25

Individualized benefits management 36

Injury
among adolescents of all ages 10
as cause of death ix, 4
comprehensive and coordinated care
63
health professionals' awareness of 50
hospitalization 10
male adolescents 54
physician visits 7
school-based health centers 23

Inpatient services (see also Hospitalization)
age differences in 14
description of 14
diagnoses 14
effectiveness of 16, 18

health expenses 38-40
health maintenance organizations
(HMOs) 32
insurance coverage xi, 16
length of stay 16
prevalence of 13, 14
psychiatric hospitalization 14, 16
race and ethnic differences in 16
sex differences in 14, 16
substance abuse treatment 18

Institute of Medicine 5

Insurance (see also Health policy, Private
insurance, Public insurance, Uninsured
adolescents) 1, 2, 27
access to care x, xi, xiii, 43, 60, 61
adequacy of x, xi, xiii, 35, 43
age differences in x, 29
alternative health care sites 21
American Academy of Family
Physicians proposal 60
American Academy of Pediatrics
proposal 60
American College of Physicians
proposal 61
American Medical Association
proposal 60
American Society of Internal Medicine
proposal 61
attitudes toward 34, 35
benefits x, 26, 43-45, 62
chronic illness 50
Civilian Health and Medical Program
of the Uniformed Services (CHAMPUS)
30
copayments 34
cost-sharing requirements 35, 60, 61
costs of 34
data on 3
disabled adolescents 50
employer-mandated health insurance
x, xii, xiii
educational status differences in 29
geographic differences in 29, 33
health care financing 58-62
health expenses 38, 40, 60, 62
hospitalization 9
income differences in xii, 29, 33, 34,
43
insured adolescents 28, 35
long-term care 61
Medicaid x, xii, xiii
Mental health services xi
parents' coverage x, xii, xiii, 28, 34
pregnancy 60
prevention and intervention 44
psychiatric hospitalization 16
public clinic use 22
race and ethnic differences in 29, 33,
43
reimbursement xi
risk pools 60
suburban adolescents 29, 33

trends in insurance status x, xii, 2, 34, 43

underinsured adolescents 59

uninsured adolescents x, 1, 28, 29, 34, 35, 43, 59, 60

Insured adolescents (see Insurance, Public insurance, Private insurance) xii, 27

Internists 8, 49, 70

Juvenile detention centers (see Incarcerated adolescents)

Koop, C. Everett 50

Legal status of adolescents 25, 51-53, 66

Local coordinating councils 64

Male adolescents
AIDS 19
alcohol 18
condoms 20
depression 54
health expenses 37
health services 54
HIV infection 19
hospitalization 9, 11, 14
injury 8, 54
mental health services 13, 54
older adolescents 8
outpatient services 13
patient-provider communication 54
reproductive health 19, 20, 54
risk-taking behavior 54
school-based health centers 23
sexually transmitted diseases 19
skin problems 8
substance abuse treatment services 18

Malocclusion 11, 12

Mandated employer-provided health insurance 59, 61, 62

Marijuana use ix

Maternal and Child Health Bureau (MCHB) 64, 67, 69

Maternity-related services (see also Reproductive health) 36, 42
abortion 20
access to care 46, 60
adoption 20
age differences in 7, 10
barriers to care 46
childbirth ix
coordinated care 47
expenses for 42
funding 59, 63
health policy 59
hospitalization 9, 10, 11
Maternal and Child Health block grants 46
Medicaid 42
office-based physicians 7
out-of-pocket expenses 40, 41
physician training 48

pregnancy xi, 20, 42, 48, 52, 59
prevalence of visits 7, 8, 20
Robert Wood Johnson Foundation 63
school-based health centers 23
Title V 46
trends in 4
use of 7, 8, 20, 46, 57

Medicaid (see Early and Periodic Screening, Diagnosis, and Treatment [EPSDT] Program, Health policy, Poverty, Public insurance)

Medical examinations 7

Medical specialists (see also specific subspecialty) 1, 2, 8

Mental health and disorders (see also specific disorders, Hospitalization, Mental health services) 1, 2, 4
age differences in ix, 10, 15
age at onset 13
alcohol and drug abuse 13, 14, 16
anxiety disorders 13
data on 15
delinquency 13
depression 16
diagnostic and testing criteria 15
disabled adolescents ix
effective treatment 16
health expenses of 37, 42
hospitalization 10, 15
incarcerated adolescents 24
insurance coverage for xi
learning disabilities 16
long-term effects of 13
neurosis 14, 15
Office of Technology Assessment 13
personality disorders 13, 14
physician training 48
prevalence of ix, 13, 15, 16
psychosis 13, 14
race and ethnic differences in 16
severity of 13
suicide 16

Mental health services 13-16
aftercare services 16
age differences in 13, 15, 41
case management 16
community-based services 14, 16
comprehensive and coordinated care xi, 16, 63
cost of 38, 39, 41
diagnosis of adolescents 15
disabled adolescents 13
Handbook on Psychiatric Practice in the Juvenile Court 68
health maintenance organizations (HMOs) 32
high-risk adolescents 63
incarcerated adolescents 25
income differences in use of 16
insurance coverage for 14, 32
juvenile courts 68

legal status of adolescents 53
need for ix, 13, 14, 16
outpatient services 13, 14, 36, 41
partial hospitalization 13, 41
physician training 68
private practice 13
psychiatric hospitalization 13, 14, 41
public insurance coverage 36
race and ethnic differences in 13, 16
reimbursement for xi
residential treatment centers (RTCs) 13, 14, 41
school-based health centers 23
sex differences in 13, 54
types of 13, 14, 41

Minority adolescents (see also Alaskan Native adolescents, Asian American adolescents, Black adolescents, Hispanic adolescents, Native American adolescents)
access to care x
alternative health care sites 21
barriers to care xiii
data on 14
dental visits 12
emergency rooms 21
health care financing 58
health policy 65
health professionals' attitudes toward 50
inpatient services 14
insurance x, 21
mental health services 14, 16
outpatient services 14
partial hospitalization 14
patient-provider communication 50
public clinics 21

National Ambulatory Medical Care Survey (NAMCS) 7

National Drug and Alcoholism Treatment Unit Survey (NDATUS) 17

National Health Interview Survey (NHIS) 3

National Institute of Mental Health (NIMH) 16

National Medical Association (NMA) 65

National Medical Care Expenditure Survey (NMCES) 38

National Medical Care Utilization and Expenditure Survey (NMCUES) 3, 38

National Medical Expenditure Survey (NMES) 38

National surveys 3, 7, 16, 38

Native American adolescents (see also Minority adolescents) 3, 16, 65

Nurses 48

Obesity 4

Obstetricians and gynecologists (see also American College of Obstetricians and Gynecologists [ACOG]) 8, 49

Office for Substance Abuse Prevention (OSAP) 64, 65

Office of Disease Prevention and Health Promotion 67

Office of Technology Assessment (OTA) 16, 18, 62

Office-based physicians 2, 7, 8, 50
    office policies of physicians 51

Older adolescents (see also Young adolescents)
    abortion 20
    definition of 2
    family planning clinics 19
    health expenses of 37, 41
    hospitalization 9, 14
    insurance coverage of 29
    maternity-related services 7
    medical specialist visits 8
    mental health services 15
    psychiatric hospitals 15
    skin problems 7

Omnibus Budget Reconciliation Act of 1989 (see also Health care financing, Health policy) 36, 37

Ophthalmologists 8

Orthodontists 12

Orthopedic surgeons 8

Out-of-pocket expenses (see also Health care financing, Health policy, Insurance) 2, 27, 38-41, 62
    access to care 60
    acute illnesses 40
    comprehensive benefits 62
    copayment requirements 40
    cost-sharing requirements 63
    deductibles 63
    disabled adolescents 42
    employer-based insurance 62
    health care financing 58, 62
    hospital services 40
    insurance 32, 40, 42, 60, 62, 63
    maternity-related services 42
    Medicaid 40, 62
    outpatient services 40
    prescription medicine 40
    preventive services 40
    rate of 39
    third-party payers 40
    uninsured adolescents 40, 41, 42

Outpatient services (see also Health services) 14
    disabled adolescents 41
    expenses for 38, 39, 40
    insurance coverage ix, 16, 36
    medical evaluation 13

mental health services 14
race differences 13
sex differences 13
types of therapy 13
use of 13, 14, 18

Parental consent/notification (see also Legal status of adolescents)
    abortion 20
    alcohol and substance abuse-related 53
    American Medical Association 65
    barriers to care 56
    contraceptive use 65
    health policy 53, 65, 66
    health services 53
    legal status of adolescents 65, 66
    mental health issues 53
    patient-provider confidentiality 65
    physician visits 52, 56, 66

Partial hospitalization 13, 14

Patient-provider communication xii, 50, 51, 55, 67

Patient-provider confidentiality xi, xiii, 1, 2, 45, 46
    abuse and neglect 51
    alcohol-related visits 52
    barriers to care xi, 46, 51, 52, 54
    contraceptives and reproductive health issues 51, 52, 65
    decision-making responsibility 65
    depression 51, 52
    health expenses 38
    health policy 65, 66
    homeless adolescents 25, 26
    legal status of adolescents 51, 52, 65, 66
    physician support for 53
    routine health care 52
    substance abuse-related visits 51, 52
    weight-related visits 52

Pediatricians 8, 37, 47, 51, 67, 70

Periodicity of health visits 5, 67

Physical disorders 1

Physician training 2, 45, 47, 49, 66-68
    adolescent medicine xi, 47, 66, 67
    adolescent sexual behavior 68
    advocacy training 68
    alcohol-related 48, 49
    benefits of 48
    chronic illness 50
    comprehensive and coordinated care 63
    depression-related 48
    disabilities 68
    drug-related 48, 49, 67
    funding of 49
    health promotion xiii, 67
    health services 46
    Healthy People 2000 68
    Healthy Youth 2000 68

improvement needed in xiii, 48, 49
Maternal and Child Health Bureau 47, 67
number of adolescent medical specialists 47-49, 67
patient-provider communication 67
pregnancy-related 48
preventive services xi, 49, 67, 68
Project Prevention 68
psychosocial problems xi, 66, 68
referral 66
Robert Wood Johnson Foundation 63
Society for Adolescent Medicine (SAM) 68
sports medicine 67
suicide-related 48

Physician visits (see also Health services) x, 2, 4, 5
    age differences in x, 5, 7, 8
    alcohol-related 52, 55
    assessment 50
    barriers to care 49, 55, 66
    confidentiality 65, 66
    content of 5
    contraceptives 7, 52, 55
    cough and throat problems 8
    counseling 50, 66
    data on 3
    depression-related 52
    dermatologists 8
    diagnoses from 7
    drug-related 52
    duration of xi, 50
    ear, nose, and throat specialists 8
    family income differences in 6
    female adolescents 8
    frequency of x, 5, 6, 67
    general and family practitioners 8
    general medical examination 7, 50, 66
    general surgeons 8
    growth-related issues 55
    guidelines for 67
    Guidelines for Adolescent Preventive Services (GAPS) 67
    health policy 65-67
    injury-related 7
    internists 8
    legal status of adolescents 66
    male adolescents 8
    maternity-related visits 7, 8, 52
    medical specialists 8
    National Ambulatory Medical Care Survey 7
    number of 5
    nutrition-related 55
    obstetricians and gynecologists 8
    Office of Disease Prevention and Health Promotion 67
    office-based physician visits 7, 8, 50
    ophthalmologists 8
    orthopedic surgeons 8
    parent-adolescent relationship 65
    parental involvement 66

patient-provider relationship 66
pediatricians 8, 67
prevalence of x, 5, 6, 7
preventive care x, 5, 7, 8, 67
primary care physicians 8
psychiatrists 8
race and ethnic differences in 6
reasons for x
recommendations for 5
referrals 50
regional differences in 6
reimbursement xi
reproductive health 7
routine office visits 52
rural adolescents 6
school-based health centers 50
sex differences in diagnoses 8
sexually transmitted diseases (STDs) 52, 55
skin problems 7, 8
substance use 55
suburban adolescents 6
throat problems 8
time restraints 49
topics discussed during 55
type of physician visited 8
uninsured adolescents x
urban and rural differences 6
urinary tract disorders 7
use patterns 5
weight-related visits 52

Poverty
access to care 30
barriers to care 30
disabled adolescents 26
health care financing 58, 59
health expenses 37, 39, 41
hospitalization rates 9
insurance status 29, 33-35
Medicaid xii, 30, 34, 35, 43
physician visits 6
uninsured adolescents x, 29, 34

Preferred provider organizations (PPOs) 32, 42

Pregnancy (see Maternity-related services, Reproductive health)

Prenatal care (see Maternity-related services, Reproductive health) 20, 42

Prescription medicine xi, 23, 36, 38, 39

Prevention and intervention (see also Health services, Health policy, Preventive care)
access to care 36
coordinated care 47
Early and Periodic Screening, Diagnosis, and Treatment (EPSDT) Program 36, 37
health expenses 37, 38
health services 26, 36, 47
health-threatening behaviors 67
high-risk adolescents 64

insurance coverage 36, 44
local coordinating councils 64
Medicaid 36
Office for Substance Abuse Prevention (OSAP) 64
physician training 67
substance abuse treatment services 18

Preventive care (see also Health services, Health policy, Prevention and intervention) 1, 3, 4
advocacy training 68
anticipatory guidance 5
assessment 5
content of visits 5, 49
coordinated care 47
dental health 11
detection of disease 5
Early and Periodic Screening, Diagnosis, and Treatment (EPSDT) Program 36
frequency of visits 5
guidelines for 5, 49
Guidelines for Adolescent Preventive Services (GAPS) 67
health education 5
health expenses 37, 38, 40
health policy 5, 67
health services 47
Institute of Medicine 5
insurance coverage xi, 36, 43
local coordinating health councils 64
Medicaid xi
mental health disorders 68
minority adolescents 43
need for 1
parental involvement 5
physician training 67, 68
physician visits x, 5, 7
prevalence of visits 7, 8
Project Prevention 68
recommendations for 5
school-based health centers 23
services recommended 5
sex differences in 8
trends in 4

Primary care (see Health services, Physician visits, Prevention and intervention, Preventive care)

Primary care physicians 8, 46, 48

Private insurance (see also Health policy, insurance, Public insurance, Uninsured adolescents) xi, 2, 43
access to care xii
acute illness 36
adequacy of xi, 35, 36
alternative setting coverage 36
among adolescents of all ages 28
benefit restrictions 35
black adolescents 33
case management xi, 36
central-city adolescents 33

characteristics of xi, 36
coinsurance 40
copayments 32
deductibles 32, 40
dental health 36
disabled adolescents 41
educational differences 33
emergency room use 36
employer-based plans xiii, 43
health care financing xii, 58, 61, 62
health maintenance organizations (HMOs) 32
health services 46
Hispanic adolescents 33
hospitalization xi
income differences in 33, 43, 60
individualized benefits management 36
living arrangement differences 33
maternity-related services xi, 36
Medicaid 34
mental health services 36
nongroup plans 32
out-of-pocket expenses 32, 40
outpatient services xi, 36
physician services xi
poverty 33
preferred provider organizations (PPOs) 32
prescription medicine 36
prevalence of x, 28, 32, 33
preventive care xi, 36
psychiatric treatment 36
regional differences 33
rural adolescents 33
school-based health clinics 36
substance abuse treatment coverage xi
suburban adolescents 33
traditional plans xi, 32
trends in 60, 61
types of 32
uninsured adolescents 35, 61
White adolescents 33

Psychiatric hospitals (see also Hospitalization, Mental health services)
adjustment reaction 15
age differences in 14, 15
alcohol abuse 15
controversy over 15, 16
cost of 42
diagnosis of adolescents 15
disturbance of conduct 15
health expenses of 42
inpatient 14
insurance coverage 16
length of stay 42
National Institute of Mental Health (NIMH) 16
neurosis 15
personality disorders 15
prevalence of 14
psychosis 15
reasons for use 16
stigma of 16

substance abuse 15
trends in 15
type of 14

Psychiatrists 8, 47

Psychologists 36, 39, 48

Public clinics 21, 22

Public insurance (see also Health policy, Insurance, Poverty, Private insurance, Uninsured adolescents) 2, 43, 59-61
access to care xi, xii, 30, 36, 46
adequacy of 30, 35, 36
age and income eligibility levels xii, 28, 30, 34, 35, 59, 60, 62
barriers to care 30, 46
benefits 30, 35, 36
black adolescents 31
case management xi, 36
characteristics of 31
Civilian Health and Medical Program of the Uniformed Services (CHAMPUS) 30
controversy over 37
coordinated care 36
definition of 30
disabled adolescents 41, 43
Early and Periodic Screening, Diagnosis, and Treatment (EPSDT) Program 36
educational differences 31
expansion for uninsured adolescents xii, xiii, 40, 60, 62
Federal poverty level xii
geographic differences 31
health services xi, 30, 46
health status of those covered by 43
Hispanic adolescents 31
income differences in 31, 35
living arrangement differences 31
Maternal and Child Health block grants 46
Medicaid x, xii, xiii, 30, 31, 35, 36, 40, 62
Medicare 30
nonphysician services coverage xi
out-of-pocket expenses 40
physician participation in Medicaid 37
poverty 30, 31
preexisting conditions 43
prevalence of x, 28, 30, 31
preventive care xi, 36
psychiatric hospitalization 36
race and ethnic differences in 31
reimbursement rates xi, 37
substance abuse treatment services xi, 36
Supplemental Security Income (SSI) 30
Title V 46
traditional medical services xi, 36
trends in coverage xiii, 34

Referral services 18

Regular source of care 43

Reproductive health (see also Contraceptive use, Family planning, Health services, Maternity-related services) 1, 2, 4, 19
clinical settings 19
contraceptive use 22
counseling 19
family planning 19, 22
female adolescents 19
health expenses 42
older adolescents 19
pregnancy testing 19
prevalence of visits 7
race differences in 19
school-based health centers 22, 23
sexual activity 19

Residential treatment centers (RTCs) (see also Health services, Mental health services, Partial hospitalization, Psychiatric hospitals) 10, 13, 14

Risk-taking behaviors (see Health-threatening behavior, High-risk adolescents)

Robert Wood Johnson Foundation 63, 69, 70

Routine health care 46

Rural adolescents xiii, 6, 9, 29, 31, 33

School-based health centers (see also Health services, Prevention and intervention, Preventive care) 2, 4, 21
controversy over 22
diagnoses made at 23
enrollment in 23
funding for 24
health education 23
length of visit 50
limitations of 24
male adolescents 23
number of 22
physician role in 24
private insurance coverage 36
regular source of care 22, 23
services offered 22, 23

Sex education 56

Sexual behavior 51, 68
abortions 19
access to care 57
AIDS 19
childbirth 19
contraceptive use 54, 57, 65
health education 69
health policy 65
HIV infection 19
legal status of adolescents 65
older adolescents 57
patient-provider confidentiality 65
pregnancy 19
prevalence of 19, 57
sex education 57
sex differences in 19, 54

sexually transmitted diseases (STDs) ix, 19, 57
trends in 54

Sexually transmitted diseases (STDs) (see also AIDS, HIV [human immunodeficiency virus] infection, Sexual behavior) ix, 1, 4, 52, 53, 55-57
access to care 57
adolescent knowledge of 56, 57
barriers to care 56
comprehensive care and coordinated care 63
health policy issues 53
parental consent/notification regarding treatment 53
patient-provider communication 55
physician visits 52, 53, 55, 56
prevalence of ix, 57
sex education 57
trends in 4

Social morbidities ix, 26

Social services (see also Comprehensive health services, Local coordinating councils) xi, 48

Society for Adolescent Medicine (SAM) 68

Substance abuse 2, 4
comprehensive care for 63
consequences of 17
coordinated care for 63
dropouts 17
Drug Abuse Warning Network (DAWN) 22
emergency room visits 22
family relations 17
female adolescents 18
health education 69
incarcerated adolescents 24
male adolescents 18
mental health and disorders 14
outpatient services 18
patient-provider communication 55
peer relations 17
physician training 48, 49
physician visits 52, 55
psychiatric hospitals 15
school performance 17
trends in 4, 17

Substance abuse treatment services (see also Hospitalization, Mental health services, Physician visits) 1, 17, 70
coordinated care xi, 47
cost of 42
data on 17
effectiveness of 18
expenses of 41
family impact on 17, 18
health expenses 37, 41
health maintenance organizations

(HMOs) 32
health services 47
inpatient services 18
insurance xi, 18, 32
marijuana use 17
National Drug and Alcoholism
Treatment Unit Survey (NDATUS) 17
need for 18
Office of Technology Assessment
(OTA) 18
out-of-pocket expenses 40
outpatient services 18
participation in 17, 18
prevention and intervention programs
18
private services 18
public services 18
referral services 18
self-help programs 18
sex differences in 18
types of 18
young adolescents 18

Suburban adolescents 6, 10, 29, 33, 52

Suicide (see also Mental health services)
ix, 4, 16, 25, 48, 50, 63

Surgeons 8

Tooth decay 11

U.S. Preventive Services Task Force 67

U.S. Public Health Service
Healthy People 2000 68
preventive care recommendations 5

Underinsured adolescents (see also Insurance, Health policy, Private
insurance, Public insurance, Uninsured
adolescents) 46, 58, 59

Uninsured adolescents (see also Health
policy, Insurance, Private insurance,
Public insurance, Underinsured
adolescents) 27
access to care x, 46
age differences in xii, 28, 29
barriers to care 46
characteristics of x, 29, 35
consequences of x, 2, 43
disabled adolescents x, 43
frequency of health care visits x, 43
geographic differences 29
health care financing 58
health care needs of 1
health policy xii, xiii, 59, 62
health services x, 46
health status x, 34, 43
hospitalization rates x, 43
income differences 29, 35
living arrangements of 29, 34
Medicaid xii, xiii, 35, 60, 62
out-of-pocket expenses x, 40, 41
parental coverage 29, 34, 62
parents' reasons for 35
poverty 29, 59

preexisting conditions 43
prevalence of x, 28, 34, 43
private insurance 60, 61
public clinics 22
race and ethnic differences 29
reasons for 34
regular source of care 43
trends in 34, 43

Violence ix, 4, 50

White adolescents
American College of Obstetricians and
Gynecologists 65
dental visits 11, 12
family planning clinics 19
health expenses 37
health policy 65
hospitalization 9
mental health services 16
older adolescents 19
outpatient mental health services 13
prevalence of insurance coverage 29
private insurance coverage 33
public clinic use 22
public insurance 31
reproductive health ix, 19

Young adolescents
definition of 2
family planning clinics 19
health expenses of 37
homicide ix
hospitalization 9
inpatient services 14
insurance coverage of 29
maternity-related services 7
medical specialist visits 8
mental health services 8, 15
suicide ix

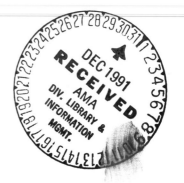